The
Complete Guide
To
Foreign Medical Schools

...In Plain English

Other Books from Indus Publishing Corporation

The Family Guide to Diseases *In Plain English*

Control Yourself
Learn how to control anger, stress, and fear and remain happy forever

The Non-Trivial Trivia Book

The Complete Guide To Foreign Medical Schools

...In Plain English

by

Nilanjan Sen

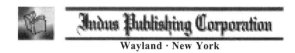

Indus Publishing Corporation

Wayland · New York

Indus Publishing Corporation
7052 Pokey Moonshine
Wayland, NY 14572
Fax: 716-728-9756

Limits of Liability and Disclaimer of Warranty:
The author and publisher have used their best efforts in preparing this book and make no warranty of any kind, expressed or implied, with regard to the instructions and suggestions contained herein. This book is only intended to be used as a reference. All advice should be obtained from competent, licensed professionals.

ISBN: 1-890838-00-4
Library of Congress: 97-093660

Credits:

The images used herein were obtained from IMSI's MasterClips Collection, 1895 Francisco Blvd. East, San Rafael, CA 94901-5506, USA.

Additional images under license from Nova Development Corporation, USA.

Cover Design: Linda Ann Scura

Manufactured in the United States of America

3 2 1

Table of Contents

Decisions, Decisions

What to do with life?

- What if you don't get into a medical school in the United States…
  …and you still want to be a doctor?

- Calm down. You can still become a doctor!

- There are lots of foreign medical schools that accept students from the United States and Canada.

- Before you decide to attend one, read this book and find out everything you need to know about foreign medical schools.

CHAPTER 1

What To Look For In Foreign Medical Schools

Foreign medical schools vary considerably in the quality of education that they provide. Some schools offer a medical education that is comparable to that of U.S. medical schools, while other schools are nothing more than a collection of small classrooms offering nothing short of an inferior education. Therefore, as a prospective foreign medical school student, you must thoroughly investigate each school before making your choice. Remember, your ultimate goal is to pass the board examinations and become eligible for residency programs in the United States.

Your investigative process should include all of the factors mentioned in this chapter. Take every action necessary to safeguard yourself against scams perpetuated by so called "medical schools" abroad. To depend entirely on the a school's brochure is foolhardy. Nor is it a good idea to depend solely on information obtained through the World Wide Web or the Internet. While Internet newsgroups dedicated to foreign medical schools may provide you with volumes of information on a particular school, the validity of those facts is questionable. Therefore, you must do more than simply rely on "official" brochure and newsgroups.

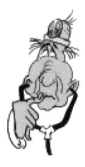

Don't worry – there are many things you can do to thoroughly evaluate the credentials of foreign medical schools. All that's required is some diligence and patience. While the best safeguard against any pitfall is to visit the campus of the foreign medical school you plan to attend, the cost of such a trip may be prohibitive. In the event you can't meake it to the campus, follow these steps to protect yourself against scams and misrepresentations by fraudulent medical schools.

Talk To Graduates

The best source of information on any foreign medical school is physicians who attended schools abroad. All reputable schools will gladly put you in contact with several graduates of their school. You should be prepared to ask them about every aspect of the medical education at their alma mater. That means you must do your homework before talking to them. Research everything about the school. Use every resource at your disposal – the Internet, brochures and flyers and your premedical advisor. Ask the big questions that will help you learn more about the school. Here are some sample questions:

■ How many students pass the USMLE Parts I and II on their first try?

■ In what types of hospitals do graduates obtain residency positions?

■ Did graduates of your school have any problem working with US trained physicians?

■ Did you experience any professional discrimination because of your foreign medical degree?

■ Where are clinical rotations held during the 3rd and 4th year of medical school?

■ What are the backgrounds and professional experiences of professors?

■ What is the quality of the laboratories and classrooms at the school?

■ What is the library like?

■ Are there any on-campus housing and dining centers?

Clinical Rotations

It is extremely important that all or a significant part of your clinical curriculum is completed in the United States. Schools that have formal clinical training programs in the U.S. are more respected by American medical institutions. Graduates from those schools tend to obtain better residencies. Some schools have their students complete their clinical rotations at their affiliated hospitals in the U.S., while other schools let their students do rotations in the U.S. *if* he or she arrange it with a hospital. If a school that you are considering has a U.S.-based clinical program, check to see if most of the affiliated hospitals where rotations will be performed are teaching or community hospitals. Since teaching hospitals tend to have residency programs, they are better equipped to train medical students and young doctors. You need all the help you can get when it comes to passing the United States Medical Licensing Examination (USMLE). Completing your clinical rotations in teaching hospitals will certainly better prepare you for your future profession as well as the USMLE.

A word of caution. In 1994, the U.S. Government Accounting Office (GAO) conducted a study and found that 61% of the hospitals that claimed to be affiliated with various Caribbean and Mexican medical schools were not formally affiliated with any foreign medical school. Of the hospitals that were affiliated, 29% did not have residency programs. However, the most astonishing fact discovered by the report was that 10% of the so-called affiliated hospitals did not exist. Usually, medical schools in Israel, Australia and Western Europe have adequate medical training facilities. Medical schools, such as St. Georges's University (Grenada), have done an impressive job of affiliating themselves with notable hospitals in both the United States and the United Kingdom. But St. George's is an exception. You should call as many hospitals as possible to verify if they are truly affiliated with the foreign medical school of your choice.

Teaching Facilities

Numerous foreign medical schools seized the opportunity to attract hundreds of U.S. citizens who were rejected by American medical schools since the number of applicants to U.S. medical schools skyrocketed in early 1990s. Unfortunately, few of the foreign schools have the resources of U.S. medical schools. Now, with hundreds of Americans heading abroad for school, the situation has only worsened.

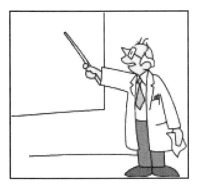

Often, the so-called campuses are nothing more than a few rooms or buildings, set up in haste, to welcome unsuspecting medical students. Often there are shortages of electricity and water on campus. Such shortages can lead to unsanitary conditions that may be detrimental to the health of the students. Lack of air-conditioning in warm weather countries (ex: Caribbean region) can make studying medicine there an uncomfortable proposition.

Many foreign schools lack libraries and computer facilities. The fast evolving world of medicine churns out information at warp speed and medical students must keep up with it. Students must be adept at using and processing information on-line. Lack of computer facilities with Internet connections may severely handicap your ability to acquire the latest medical news. Furthermore, lack of current medical periodicals and journals at a school library will also hinder the progress of your study.

Finally, the state of the anatomy laboratory should be of prime concern to you. Much of your first year will be spend inside the anatomy laboratory. Insufficient numbers of cadavers and crowded conditions inside the laboratory will adversely affect your education. It is extremely important for you to find out the average number of students assigned to each cadaver at a given school. Typically, the U.S. medical schools assign four students to each cadaver.

In summary, you must thoroughly investigate the physical facilities of all foreign medical schools prior to matriculating at one.

Residency Appointments

The two factors that have the greatest impact on the residency-matching process are your USMLE scores and the reputation of the school that you attend. Residency directors and hospital administrators are often unenthusiastic about offering position to graduates of foreign medical schools they are not aware of. Graduates of better medical schools find it easier to get into the more desirable residency programs. Ask medical schools for a list of hospitals where recent graduates were accepted to complete their residencies. Once you have obtained the list, randomly contact the hospitals to verify the validity of the list.

Faculty

Foreign medical schools often inflate the qualifications of their faculty. A large number of them claim that some of their faculty members were former professors at US medical schools and universities. Furthermore, a handful of schools claim certain professors as part of their permanent faculty even though he or she only taught at the school for a semester during a previous year. When evaluating a foreign medical school, thoroughly scrutinize the background of the senior faculty.

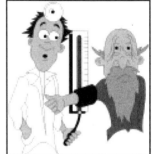

Also, if you are interested in attending a medical school in a non-English speaking country, verify the English proficiency of the professors. Even if the professors have a working knowledge of the English language, their heavy accents may hinder your comprehension. Be prepared to deal with such situations.

Life Outside the Campus

Living abroad during your medical school years is an unique experience. However, you may well attend medical school in a country whose living standards are inferior to that of American living standards. The availability of fresh groceries and a ready supply of electricity will vary greatly from country to country. Everyday amenities, such as guaranteed telephone service, may not be the norm in your host country. You must be prepared to compromise and make the best of the situation. In addition, laws of other nations are different from U.S. laws. You must be aware of local traditions and customs in order to peacefully live in a foreign community.

While a few schools make a sincere effort assisting their students in successfully integrating into local communities, most foreign medical schools do not have the resources nor money to commit to such programs. Living conditions are important for your mental health. If you are dissatisfied with your life in a foreign country, it will be extremely difficult to do well in medical school. So, be meticulous in your research when it comes to living abroad and the life-style that is associated with it.

Curriculum and Textbooks

Any reputable foreign medical school will follow a similar curriculum to that of U.S. medical schools. In addition, a good foreign medical school should also use standard textbooks that are well-known and respected. Check with current U.S. medical students for the names of standard medical school textbooks used in U.S. schools. You may also consider contacting U.S. medical schools for their first and second year class book list.

Be aware that a handful of foreign medical schools offer "accelerated" three year programs. No U.S. medical school offers a medical program that is shorter than four years. As a result, three year curriculums are not considered to be on the same par as four year programs. Conversely, a few Eastern European schools offer a M.D. program that lasts approximately five or six years. These programs combine both undergraduate and graduate medical studies in an unified curriculum. If you already possess an undergraduate degree, you may consider staying away from any M.D. program that lasts for more than four years.

Financial Aid

Matriculating at a medical school is an expensive proposition. Before you commit $100,000 to a foreign school, inquire about its financial stability. You certainly do not want to loose money half way through your medical education when your school suddenly decides to permanently shut down. A majority of the schools abroad are not eligible for U.S. Federal Government sponsored loan programs. A good sign of financial stability is a school's eligibility for US Federal loans. Make sure to check with the U.S. Department of Education whenever a foreign medical school claims to be eligible for U.S. Federal loans.

CHECK LIST – MEDICAL SCHOOL INQUIRY

- **Talk to graduates**
- **Inquire about the location of clinical rotations**
- **Inquire about teaching facilities**
- **Inquire about recent residency appointments**
- **Inquire about the faculty's background**
- **Inquire about life outside the medical school**
- **Inquire about the curriculum and textbooks**
- **Inquire about the financial stability of the school**

Financial Aid

What You *Need* To Know

CHAPTER 2

Financial Aid
What You Need To Know

There is no doubt that foreign medical schools are just as expensive as American medical schools when it comes to tuition and fees. For the 1996-97 school year, the average first-year tuition at private U.S. medical schools was just over $25,000. Foreign medical school tuition was not too far behind the U.S. schools. In addition, added costs, such as traveling back and forth between a foreign nation and the United States, can make attending a medical school abroad a very expensive proposition. Unfortunately, an overwhelming majority of foreign medical schools do not offer financial aid packages that are grant based. Furthermore, only a few of the foreign medical schools are eligible for loan programs sponsored by the U.S. Federal Government. As a result, either you or your family must be able to pay all of the costs of attending medical school or find alternate sources of funding, such as private loan programs, to finance your medical education.

A Word of Caution!

A large number of medical schools have been set up to lure American students to destinations all over the world. Most of them are nothing more than fronts to collect money from students who are desperately seeking to study medicine. As a potential applicant to a foreign medical school, you must be aware of scams at all times. Your skills to detect scams will best be tested when it comes to understanding the complex world of financial aid and foreign medical schools. It is important to note that there are many reputable foreign medical schools such as St. George's (Grenada), Ross University (Dominica) and Sackler School of Medicine (Israel) that maintain fully-staffed financial aid offices to truly assist students in financial need. You must watch out for the exceptions.

So what must you do to determine whether a school's financial aid division is legitimate or not? There are two things you should look for. First, all reputable schools should have financial aid counselors who can give you detailed information about the financial aid process including the types of loan programs available to eligible students. Make sure that counselors who advise you are **not** working as admissions agents for the school. Rather, they are employed by the medical school's financial aid division.

Second, if a school says that its students are eligible for Federal Loan Programs (such as the Stafford Loan), ask for the school's United States Department of Education code number. Without a code number, a school is not eligible for Federal Loan Programs. Once you obtain the code, contact a major bank's student loan division to verify the code number and the school's eligibility.

Financial Aid Programs

There are two types of financial assistance available to students: *loans* and *scholarships.* Except for a few schools, most do not offer academic scholarships. Academic scholarships or grants provide money that does not have to be repaid. In other words, it is free. Since most foreign medical schools do not operate on large budgets, they cannot offer scholarships or loans. They do offer a few privately-sponsored scholarships to students who have demonstrated academic excellence. However, a vast majority of foreign medical schools depend on loans as the primary form of financial assistance for students in need.

Loans

Loans must be repaid to the lender. The lender may be a governmental or private agency or the medical school itself. All loans are repaid with interests. Usually, U.S. Government loans have lower interest rates than do most privately-sponsored loan programs. In order to qualify for federal loan programs, certain criteria must be met. However, the most important factor is whether or not the foreign medical school you would like to attend is eligible for Federal Loan programs.

There are *four* types of loans: federal, state, private and institutional.

> **Financial Aid & Foreign Medical Schools: What to Look For**
>
> Just because a school participates in the Federal Loan Program does not mean the U.S. Department of Education endorses the quality of the education the school offers. In fact, the Department does not approve a school's curriculum, policies, or administrative practices. It's up to you to check out the school. Ask the schools the following questions:
>
> - Ask to see the school's copy of the documents describing its accreditation and licensing.
>
> - Ask the school about its loan default rate.
>
> - Ask the school for its graduation rate.
>
> - Ask the school about its tuition refund policy.

Federal: Federal loan programs are funded by the federal government. Most federal loans are need based. All federal loan programs have a maximum amount that students can borrow in a given year. Federal loans also tend to have the lowest interest rates in comparison to any other type of loan.

State: State loans are only extended to students who attend medical schools in a particular U.S. state. Since all foreign medical school are chartered outside the U.S., students attending schools abroad are not eligible for any state loans.

Private: Private loans are funded by foundations, religious organizations, fraternities or sororities, community organizations and civic groups like YMCA, Kiwanis, or 4-H Club. Most private loans are targeted at specific segments of the population such as disadvantaged students or women. Interest rates and repayment plans of private loans vary greatly. It is important to perform thorough research on lending organizations before applying for private loans from them.

Institutional: On rare occasions schools extend loans to a student to cover that student's expenses. Do not expect institutional loans from any school since most of them are working within tight budget constraints.

Scholarships

Scholarships or grants do not need to be repaid, but that does not mean that all grants come with no strings attached. For example, in return for free money the endowing organization may oblige you to perform a specific service for a given length of time. It is important to note that grants are not necessarily need based. Often families and foundations establish scholarship funds targeting a specific demographic group. For instance, organizations like labor unions have created many grant programs for the dependents of their members.

Federal Stafford Loans

Federal Stafford Loans (Stafford Loans) are the U.S. Department of Education's major form of financial aid and are available through the Federal Direct Loan (Direct Loan) Program and the Federal Family Education Loan (FFEL) Program. The terms and conditions of a Direct Stafford or an FFEL Stafford are similar. The major differences between the two are the source of the loan funds, some aspects of the application process, and the available repayment plans. An increasing number of schools are participating in the Direct Loan Program. Under this program, the funds for Stafford Loan come directly from the U.S. Government. If a school does not participate in the Direct Loan Program, then the funds are forwarded from a bank or other lender that participates in the FFEL Program.

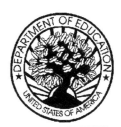

U.S.
Department of
Education
insignia

Types of Stafford Loans

Stafford Loans are either subsidized or unsubsidized. A *subsidized* loan is awarded on the *basis of financial need*. The federal government pays interest on or subsidizes the loan until a student begin repayment and during authorized periods of deferment.

An *unsubsidized* loan is *not* awarded on the *basis of financial need*. Students are charged interest from the time the loan is disbursed until it is paid in full. If the interest is allowed to accumulate, it will be capitalized – that is, interest will be added to the principal amount of the loan, increasing the amount that has to be repaid.

It is possible to receive both a subsidized and an unsubsidized Stafford Loan for the same enrollment period.

How Much Can You Borrow?

> As a medical student, you may borrow up to $18,500 each academic year. At least $10,000 of this amount must be in unsubsidized Stafford Loans.

How to Apply for a Direct Stafford Loan

All borrowers must fill out the *Free Application for Federal Student Aid (FAFSA).* After your *FAFSA* is processed, school(s) will review the results and will inform you of your loan eligibility.

You may request a *FAFSA* form by writing to this following address:

Federal Student Aid Information Center
P.O. Box 84
Washington, DC 20044

The *FAFSA* application is free and it does not cost any money to apply for federal loan programs. However, if you are approved for a loan a fee of up to four percent (4%) is deducted from the total disbursement of your loan.

If you need answers to questions about federal student aid, you can call the following number at the Federal Student Aid Information Center between 9:00 a.m. and 8 p.m. (Eastern Time), Monday through Friday:

1-800-4-FED-AID (1-800-433-3243)

How to Apply for an FFEL Stafford Loan

Follow the same procedure as for Direct Stafford Loan but remember the U.S. Government is not the lender. In this case, the lenders are institutions like banks and credit unions. Lenders can be found by contacting the guaranty agency *(see "Important Terms" section at the end of this chapter)* that serves your state. For the agency's address and telephone number, and for more information about borrowing, call the Federal Student Aid Information Center's toll-free number: 1-800-433-3243. The terms under which FFEL Stafford Loan are granted are the same as the terms related to Direct Stafford Loan.

Private Loan Programs

International Health Education Loan Program (IHELP)

IHELP was designed to offer supplemental loans to independent students. The program offers a loan package which includes the FFELP loans and a supplemental loan. The FFELP loan portion is administered in accordance with U.S. federal regulations and is described in the previous section. The supplemental loan provides additional funding. The interest rates of the loans are *higher* than those of federal loans.

The supplemental program offers loans in amounts up to the cost of attendance (or $15,000 per academic year, whichever comes first). No co-signer nor sponsor is required for U.S. students, and there is only minimal credit criteria. In some cases, non-U.S. students who have creditworthy U.S. sponsors may receive these loans as well. The interest is a variable rate based upon the 91-day T-bill plus 3.5%. There is no cap. In addition, the student pays a 10.5% guarantee fee. The repayment period of up to 20 years may begin after medical residency. Payment of both principal and interest may be deferred until repayment.

The IHELP program is administered by International Education Finance Company (IEFC), a division of Education Funding Services, Inc. (EFS). EFS, founded in 1992, has become a recognized leader in developing innovative education credit programs for various health professions on both a national and international basis. The lender for the IHELP program is BAC International Credit Corp., located in Miami, Florida.

For more information, call IEFC at 1-800-252-2041.

IHELP Loan Credit Criteria

- Credit bureau reports are obtained for each applicant.

- There is no more than one retail account 60 days late or one bank account 30 days late at the time of credit report.

- There is no account which has been delinquent 90 or more days in the past two years.

- There is no record of foreclosure, repossession, open judgment or suit, unpaid tax lien, etc.

- There is no record of bankruptcy in the past ten years.

- Borrower must be a U.S. citizen or legal resident of the United States.

Extra-Credit/Extra-Time Loan Program

The Extra Credit/Extra-Time Loan Program was designed to provide loans to the parents (or sponsors) of students who plan to attend medical school. The program provides a loan package that includes FFELP loans as well as a supplemental loan in amounts up to the cost of attendance (or $25,000 per academic year, whichever comes first). The FFELP loan portion is administered in accordance with U.S. federal regulations and described in the previous section. The supplemental program's interest rates are higher than those of federal loans. The interest is a variable rate based on the 91-

day T-bill plus 4.5%. Repayment of principal and/or interest takes place while the student is in school. The Extra-Credit borrower pays no guarantee fee and pays monthly principal and interest payments. The Extra-Time borrower pays a 3% guarantee fee and monthly interest-only payments.

Extra-Credit Loans are made available nationally through the COLLEGECREDIT education loan program, a service of the College Board.

The guidelines for these private education loan programs are subject to program changes made by the lending companies.

For more information contact:

ExtraCredit Loans
c/o Knight College Resource Group
855 Boylston Street
Boston, MA 02116-9854

1-800-874-9390

Getting Back Into The U.S.

What You *Need* To Do To Obtain Residency Position in the U.S.

CHAPTER 3

Getting Back Into The United States

The successful completion of all parts of the examinations sponsored by the Educational Commission for Foreign Medical Graduates (ECFMG) is required of all students who seek an ACGME approved postgraduate residency training program within the United States. In 1992, a new physician licensing track, the United States Medical Licensing Examination, was put in place.

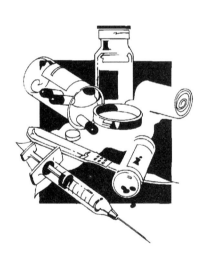

National Resident Matching Program
The function of the National Resident Matching Program (NRMP) is to match applicants seeking postgraduate residency positions in the United States with institutions offering those positions. Students are given the opportunity, as late as their senior year, to rank preferences confidentially. They are matched to the highest ranked training program on their list, which offers prospective graduate positions.

Students and graduates of foreign medical schools may enroll as individuals in the NRMP. They will be retained in the program if they submit proof of having passed the examinations required to obtain the ECFMG certification by the date of submission of rank order lists in January of each year. ECFMG certification must be obtained before beginning residency training. A non-U.S. citizen who intends to enter the U.S. as an exchange visitor must also be able to qualify under the conditions of applicable United States laws.

Information and materials may be obtained from:

National Resident Matching Program
One American Plaza – Suite 807
Evanston, IL 60201

The United States Medical Licensing Examination

The USMLE

The United States Medical Licensing Examination is a three step, multiple choice exam that must be passed by all medical school graduates, (foreign or domestic), who wish to practice medicine in the United States. The three steps are:

Step I: Basic Sciences – should be taken after completion of first two years of medical school.

Step II: Clinical Sciences – should be taken after graduation and full licensure as a doctor.

Step III: The Unsupervised Practice of Medicine – requirements vary from state to state.

The USMLE also includes an English test for all doctors trained outside the U.S., Canada and Puerto Rico. This is usually given with Step II, but may be taken separately. This test is also administered by the ECFMG.

Be sure to check if you are eligible to sit for the exams. The best sources of information are the official USMLE and ECFMG web sites.

Step I and Step II

You must pass Steps I and II before you can obtain a postgraduate medical position in the U.S. IMGs (International Medical Graduates) should write to the following address for detailed information and application papers:

ECFMG
3624 Market Street
4th floor
Philadelphia, Pennsylvania 19104-2685
USA
http://www.ecfmg.org/

The ECFMG (Educational Commission for Foreign Medical Graduates) handles all IMG applications for Steps I and II of the USMLE, including the English test.

U.S. and Canadian medical school graduates apply through their medical schools in their respective countries.

Step III

Step III is not essential for getting an internship, but it does help. However, it is usually difficult as Step III exams are given in the state in which you wish to have a license. Most states require international medical graduates to have previous experience in an accredited U.S. or Canadian program before letting them sit for Step III of the USMLE. However the following states permit IMGs take Step III without any medical training in North America (although you till have to take the exam in that state):

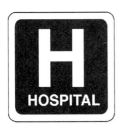

1. California

2. Connecticut

3. Maryland

4. Minnesota

5. Nebraska

6. Nevada

7. New York

8. Puerto Rico

Passing all three steps does not guarantee a medical license. Each state has its own requirements and should be contacted individually. The ECFMG booklet usually has the addresses of State Medical Licensing Boards. The deadline for applying for Step III varies widely from state to state. In addition, each state has a set of documents that it requires. Consult the Green book for more details. General inquires for Step III of the USMLE may be directed to the Federation of State Medical Boards of the United States:

FSMB
400 Fuller Wiser Road
Suite 300
Euless, Texas 76039-3855
USA
Tel: (817) 868-4000
Fax: (817) 868-4098
http://www.fsmb.org/

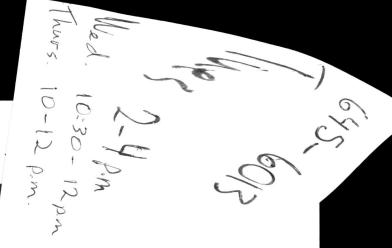

The Educational Commissi
Foreign Medical Graduates

In recognition and fulfillment of public respons
health care, its delivery, and health profession
organizations established the Educational Comm
Graduates (ECFMG).

- The American Board of Medical Specialties
- The American Hospital Association
- The American Medical Association
- The Association of American Medical Colleges
- The Association for Hospital Medical Education
- The Federation of State Medical Boards of the United States, Inc.
- The National Medical Association

The ECFMG, a non-profit organization, has the responsibility of evaluating qualifications of graduates of foreign medical schools who seek postgraduate medical education positions in the United States.

To meet its responsibilities, ECFMG identifies the following as its mission:

- To provide information to graduates of foreign medical schools regarding entry into graduate medical education and health care systems in the United States;

- To evaluate the qualifications of graduates of foreign medical schools for entry into graduate medical education and health care systems in the United States;

- To identify the cultural and professional needs of graduates of foreign medical schools and to assist in the establishment of educational policies and programs to meet these needs;

- To provide international access to testing and evaluation programs;

- To gather, maintain, analyze, and disseminate data and to conduct research studies on such data concerning graduates of foreign medical schools;

- To assist foreign medical schools and other institutions and international agencies concerned with health professions education through consultation and cooperation relative to program development, standard setting, and evaluation.

Ordering an Information Booklet:

Students and graduates of foreign medical schools interested in applying for ECFMG certification should request a copy of the combined USMLE Bulletin of Information/ECFMG Information Booklet (Form 100-S). Applicants should be sure to obtain the most current information booklet and application form (that which pertains to the examination administration for which they plan to register). Information Booklet packets include an application for USMLE Step I and Step II and the ECFMG English test.

* Telephone requests for a single copy of the Information Booklet may be made 24 hours per day, 7 days per week.

ECFMG
3624 Market Street
Philadelphia, PA 19104-2685

Fax: 215-387-9963
Phone: 215-386-5900

National Residency Matching Program

The Match

The Match is the system by which doctors and hospitals choose each other. Medical students make a list of the residency programs they are interested in. They list the programs in order of preference, from most preferred to least preferred. The hospitals make a list of candidates they would like to admit into their training programs. Both lists are submitted to the NRMP. The NRMP uses a computer to match medical students to programs by comparing their choices.

Please note, some specialty programs have their own, independent "match" programs, which have a separate application process. Also, it is possible to apply for some programs over the Internet .

Independent applicants, such as IMGs, should write to the NRMP by June of the year in which they plan to enter the program. The NRMP sends the applicant forms for joining the Match. The applicant must return the form to the NRMP by the specified Independent Application Agreement deadline.

International medical graduates need to pass Step I and II of the USMLE as well as the English test. Their credentials are verified by the ECFMG. They are then issued an ECFMG certificate which is necessary for participation in the Match.

U.S. and Canadian medical students usually apply through their medical school.

The universal application form is very useful for contacting programs, since most programs accept this form. In addition, some programs will want you to fill out their own forms. The procedure varies from program to program. It is a good idea to mail your applications by the end of June, although the deadline is in October. Remember, it takes time for your applications to reach the programs and there are a limited number of interview slots. The earlier you send out applications, the better your chances of being interviewed.

After choosing programs of interest to you, enter them on the Match form and submit it by the deadline. Always allow time for mail delays and application processing. More details can be found in the NRMP booklet "Handbook for Independent Applicants," which is enclosed with their application form.

As of June 1st, 1996 the NRMP's new address is :

National Resident Matching Program
2501 M Street , NW , Suite 1
Washington , DC 20037 - 1307
Phone: (202) 828-0566
http://www.aamc.org/about/progemph/nrmp/start.html

The Best of the Bunch

Grenada
West Indies

The Country Fact Box
GRENADA

- *Capital:* St. George's
- *Government:* Parliamentary Democracy
- *Head of Government:* Prime Minister
- *Population:* 95,000
- *Primary Languages:* English & French
  patois
- *Monetary Unit:* East Caribbean Dollar

St. George's University
School of Medicine

St. George

St. George's University
School of Medicine

Office of Admissions • C/O Medical School Services, Ltd.
One East Main Street • Bay Shore • NY 11706-8399
Phone: 516-665-8500 or 1-800-899-6337
Fax: (516) 665-5590
Email: sgu_info@sgu.edu • Internet: http://www.stgeorgesuniv.edu/univ/

St. George's University School of Medicine was founded in Grenada, West Indies in 1976. Since its inception 21 years ago, the school has granted over 2,000 M.D. degrees to qualified medical students. Graduates of St. George's now practice medicine in more than 19 countries, in all specialties and subspecialities. The current student body at the medical school is a diverse collection of international scholars hailing from such countries as the United States, the United Kingdom, India, Ireland, and Kuwait. In fact, the official St. George's brochure, published by the University, claims that there are more than 55 countries represented on campus. In addition to a diverse student body, the medical school also boasts an international professor pool.

St. George's University School of Medicine is listed in World Health Organization's *World Directory of Medical Schools*. It is also recognized and authorized by the Government of Grenada to grant Doctor of Medicine (M.D.) degrees to competent students who have successfully passed all phases of the medical school's curriculum. Furthermore, St. George's medical program is approved by the states of California, New Jersey and New York for clinical training of its students in affiliated hospitals located in those states. The medical school has also received Limited Registration status with the General Medical Council of Great Britain.

Grenada, West Indies

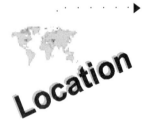

The basic sciences campuses of St. George's are located on the islands of Grenada and St. Vincent and the Grenadines in the Caribbean.

The island of Grenada is located 90 miles off the shore of Venezuela (South America). Grenada is 2,300 miles southeast of New York City and 450 miles south of Puerto Rico. The True Blue and Grand Anse basic sciences campuses are located on the southeast edge of this small island.

The island of St. Vincent, home to the Kingstown Medical College (a St. George's affiliate), is located 75 miles north of Grenada in the Caribbean basin.

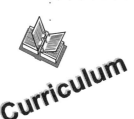

Curriculum

The Medical Program

The M.D. program at St. George's is designed to be completed in four calendar years. The medical curriculum is divided into five academic years, each lasting anywhere between 30 to 34 weeks. The total length of the program is 157 weeks.

Of the 157 weeks, the first 77 weeks (two calendar years) are spent on the islands of Grenada and St. Vincent. During this period, students matriculate in the basic science program which concentrates on the traditional medical science disciplines. Through a combination of class lectures, small-group discussions, computer-assisted instructions and laboratory sessions, the basics of fundamental sciences are conveyed to students.

The next 80 weeks of the program are clinically oriented. Students spend most of their time working in university affiliated hospitals. During the first 46 of the 80 weeks, students enter clinical rotations in departments of medicine, surgery, obstetrics/gynecology (OB/GYN), psychiatry, and pediatrics. The remaining 34 weeks are targeted for subinternships in departments of pediatrics, medicine and primary care medicine. Students may also choose to enroll in elective rotations during this period. All clinical rotations are completed at St. George's affiliated hospitals in the Caribbean, the United Kingdom, and the U.S. *(the list of affiliated hospitals is published below).*

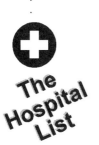

The Hospital List

The Official Clinical Affiliation List

CARIBBEAN
Grenada General Hospital
Kingstown Medical College

UNITED KINGDOM
Ashford Hospital
Barnet General Hospital
Bedford General Hospital
Chelsea & Westminister Hospitals
Edgeware General Hospital
Kent & Canterbury Hospital
Luton & Dunstable Hospital
Norfolk & Norwich Hospital
North Middlesex Hospital
James Paget Hospital
Princess Margaret Hospital
Princess Royal Hospital
Royal Naval Haslar Hospital
Royal United Hospital
St. Anne's Hospital
Stafford General Hospital
University College London

UNITED STATES
Brooklyn Hospital
Coney Island Hospital
Interfaith Medical Center
Jamaica Hospital
Maimonides Medical Center
Manhattan Psychiatric Center
Mt. Vernon Hospital
VA Medical Center
Methodist Hospital
Atlantic City Medical Center
St. Elizabeth Hospital
St. Joseph's Hospital & Med. Center
St. Michael's Medical Center
United Hospital Medical Center
Highland General Hospital
Napa State Hospital
San Joquin General Hospital
Harbor Hospital Center
Maryland General Hospital
Prince George's Hospital Center
Spring Grove Hospital Center

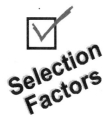

Minimum Admission Requirements

The minimum admission requirements for applicants from North America (the United States and Canada) are the following:

- A bachelor's degree from an accredited university or college prior to matriculation into the University.
- Completion of premedical curriculum that includes the following courses:
    1. General biology with laboratory – one year (two semesters)
    2. Inorganic chemistry with laboratory – one year (two semesters)
    3. Organic chemistry with laboratory – one year (two semesters)
    4. Physics with laboratory – one semester
    5. Mathematics (calculus, computer science or statistics) – one year (two semesters)
    6. English – one semester
- Medical College Admission Test (MCAT) score

Selection Factors

According to the official University brochure, the selection of students "… is made after careful consideration of many aspects: academic ability, emotional and professional maturity, academic achievement, community service, indicators of responsibility and motivation, MCAT scores when applicable, health professions' experience, and letters of recommendation…" It is important to note that the admissions committee does not rank the various selection factors in any order of importance.

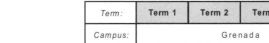

Tuition & Fees

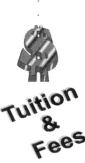

Term:	Term 1	Term 2	Term 3	Term 4	Term 5	Term 6
Campus:	Grenada				St. Vincent	
Pre-clinical	$9,307	$9,307	$3,495	$9,307	$3,495	$6,993
Fees	$2,007	$2,007	$667	$2,007	$667	$1,331

Term	Term 7	Term 8	Term 9	Term 10	Term 11
Clinicals	$9,367	$9,367	$9,367	$9,367	$9,368
Fees	$1,525	$1,525	$1,525	$1,525	$1,525
Malpractice Insurance	$ 320				
Oral Exam Fee	$ 545				
Graduation Fee	$ 292				

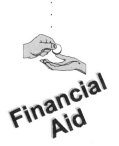

Financial Aid

Most students attending medical school at St. George's University receive some form of financial aid. The Financial Aid Services division of the University assists students with financial planning and budgeting. The vast majority of the financial aid packages received by students are in the form of loans. St. George's University is eligible for both governmental and private loans in the United States and Canada. The University also provides a small number of partial scholarships through its Institutional Aid Program.

- *Government Loan Programs (U.S. Students only):*
  1. The Subsidized Federal Stafford program – $8,500 per year
  2. The Unsubsidized Federal Stafford program – $10,000 per year

- *Private Educational Loan Programs:*
  1. Extra Credit/Extra-Time Loan Program
  2. International Health Education Loan Program

- *Institutional Aid Programs (U.S. Students only):*
  1. Congress of Italian American Organization Scholarship
  2. Geoffrey H. Bourne Scholarship
  3. Masonic Order Scholarship
  4. Graham Belz, Michael Brooker and Randall Gunther Memorial Scholarships
  5. Stephen R. Kopycinski Memorial Scholarship

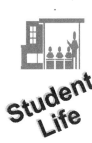

Student Life

At the time of the printing of this book, the University had two campuses on the island of Grenada and one campus on the neighboring island of St. Vincent and the Grenadines. However, a massive building process is underway in Grenada with the aim to consolidate the two campuses, the True Blue and Grand Anse, into one integrated campus.

- *Main Buildings On Campus:*
  1. The Geoffrey Bourne Lecture Hall complex
  2. Department of Physiology Building
  3. Department of Educational Science Building
  4. The Research Institute
  5. The Marion Library
  6. The New Library Building *(under construction)*
  7. The Student Center *(under construction)*

■ *Housing On Campus:*
All first-semester students are required to live on-campus. Housing on-campus is plenty and relatively comfortable. All the newer dormitories are equipped with central air-conditioning. Air-conditioning is available as an option in the older dormitories. Students may reside in off-campus apartments after the completion of their first term at Grenada. Students report that off-campus housing is satisfactory and affordable.

During the fifth and sixth-terms students are required to live in University housing on St. Vincent. The St. Vincent dormitory facilities are equipped with a laundry room, dining room and a library.

■ *Student Organizations*
1. American Medical Students Association (AMSA) of the American Medical Association
2. Iota Epsilon Alpha Honor Society
3. Emergency Medical Club
4. The Significant Others (SOs) Group
5. The Canadian Student Association

■ *Life Outside The Campus*
Students report that "the equatorial sun has a tendency to mellow human beings." In other words, life in Grenada does not take on the same type of urgency that is usually found in the United States. Some of you may look at this as something attractive, while the rest of you may be turned-off by the slow nature of life in Grenada. The recommendation from the students is simple: "You will be much happier if you go with the flow. Expect delays and be mentally prepared to deal with them."

Grenada is a typical Caribbean island full of "photo ops". Nature lovers will find the dramatic mountains and lush tropical vegetation ideal for photography. In addition, Grenada is home to some of the most magnificent white sand beaches in the world. St. George's students take full advantage of the surrounding reefs and colorful sea life by exploring them during their free time. The beautiful natural trails of the Grand Etang National Forest await those of you who enjoy hiking and sight-seeing.

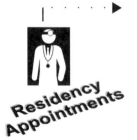

Recent Residency Appointments

The following list is a sample of various residency programs entered by graduating members of the Class of 1996:

Internal Medicine
Lenox Hill Hospital, NYC
Memorial Medical Center, GA
St. Michael's Hospital, NJ
UMDNJ Univ Hospital, NJ
Methodist Hospital, Brooklyn

Albany Medical Center, NY
Brooklyn Hospital Center, NY
Hahnemann Univ Hospital, PA
Beekman Downtown Hospital, NYC
Alameda County Medical Cntr, CA
New York Hospital, NYC

Long Island Jewish Med. Center, NY
Hennepin County Med Center, MN
Robert Byrd Health Science Cntr, WV
Beth Israel Medical Center, NYC
West Virginia Univ Hospital, WV
Univ of Connecticut Hospital, CT

Pediatrics
Children's Hospital of Oklahoma, OK
St. Luke's-Roosevelt Hospital, NYC
Univ of Florida Hospital, FL
St. Joseph's Hospital, NJ
New York Medical College, NY
Univ of Virginia Medical Center, VA
St. Joseph's Mercy Hospital, MI
Pitt Co Memorial Hospital, NC
Long Island Jewish Med. Center, NY
Monmouth Medical Center, NJ

Emergency Medicine
Beth Israel Medical Center, NYC
Brooklyn Hospital Center, NY

Family Practice & OB/GYN
St. Joseph's Hospital, NJ
Kingston Hospital, NY
Niagara Falls Mem Med. Center, NY
Southside Hospital, NY
Hamot Medical Center, PA
New Shore Univ Hospital, NY
Wayne StateUniversity. MI

General Surgery
St. Vincent's Hospital, NYC
Santa Barbara Cottage Hospital, CA
Brooklyn Hospital Center, NY
Providence Hospital, MI
St. Mary's Hospital, CT
UMDNJ Medical Center, NJ
Drew Medical Center, CA

Neurology & Anesthesiology
George Washington Univ Hospital,
Washington DC
Univ of S. Florida Med Clinics, FL

> June 1996
> USMLE Step I
> Pass Rate:
> **88.1%**

The Daily Guide

Attending medical school classes are only a part of your life in Grenada. Even in the sunny Caribbean, you will still need to use your hair dryer, listen to music or shop for food. The daily survival guide below, lists some of the useful information you need to know about life in Grenada.

Phone Calls Home
USA Direct Lines – Dial 872 (only from coin-operated *Grentel* phones)

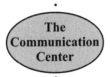

The Communication Center

Postal Service
Regular air-mails from Grenada to US require .75 EC cents and postcards require .40 EC cents. FEDEX service is available from Grenada.

Fax Service
The Grenada Student Government Copy Center provides FAX services to students. Students are charged a minimal fee for the service.

Food & Supermarkets
In the central market square, local vendors sell fresh fruits and vegetables. However, if you yearn for food imported from the U.S. you will have to go to local supermarkets. Words of warning from current students: "stores are unpredictable in terms of their inventory."

Electricity Check !!!
Grenada's electrical supply is 220 volts and 50 hertz.

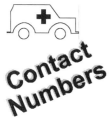

Contact Numbers

In Case Of Emergency

US Embassy
Phone#s:
(809) 444-1173/74/75/76/77/78

Grenadian Embassy (in Washington, D.C.)
Phone#: (202) 265-2561

Dean of Student Office (Grenada)
Phone#: (809) 444-3377/4483

General Statement of University Mission And Goals

St. George's University is an international center for higher education with the following goals:

- To improve health standards and health-care delivery systems throughout the world, particularly in developing countries such as Grenada, St. Vincent, and other Caribbean nations.
- To promote research in health-care related fields and preventive medicine, particularly into the causes, prevalence, or incidence, and the treatment of diseases important to communities in the Windward Islands and the greater Caribbean.
- To prepare competent students for the practice of medicine in the public and private sectors with the skills essential for improving existing health-care delivery systems, thereby promoting the highest goals of the medical profession.

In Their Own Words...

Comments From The Staff Of St. George's

General Statement From The Dean Of Enrollment Planning

St. George's University School of Medicine (SGUSOM) is a highly competitive medical school which trains physicians to practice medicine in today's world. There are approximately 8-9 applicants for each seat in the Medical School. The average undergraduate GPA is 3.4; the average composite MCAT is 26. Our Board of Admissions selects students, not only for their mastery of the necessary academic foundation, but also for their experience in the health field, experience living abroad, and demonstrated commitment to the community.

The School is committed to academic excellence. The pass rate on the June 1996 USMLE I for first time takers was 88.1%; the worldwide pass rate on the USMLE I hovers around 55%. The curriculum is constantly being reviewed and revised to reflect changes in medicine and educational theory. The material is delivered in a multi-faceted approach which includes traditional lectures and laboratories, as well as small group sessions with problem-based learning. The Clinical Skills course begins in the first term with small groups in outlaying clinics on the island of Grenada and continues throughout the basic sciences years. This clinical training is completed at our affiliated hospitals in the United States and the United Kingdom.

Over 2,400 physicians have graduated from SGUSOM, most of whom are in community or academic medicine in the United States. Just recently, the U.S. Department of Education reviewed the accreditation process for medical schools of 30 countries whose medical schools enroll U.S. students. This was done to ensure that U.S. government sponsored loans would go to students enrolled in only those schools whose standards are deemed comparable to U.S. medical schools; only those that, in the words of the U.S. Secretary of Education, Richard W. Riley, "provide a high quality education to its students." As of April, 1997, Grenada is one of only four countries that have currently met this criteria. The other countries are Australia, Canada and the United Kingdom.

SGUSOM provides students with an excellent education in a multi-cultural environment. Our mission has changed in the past 10 years. We are now dedicated to becoming a truly international School of Medicine with more than 50% international student enrollment. Our goal is to train students from countries that need physicians; they will return to their home counries where they are much needed. The last academic year saw an influx of 20% international students. 55 countries are represented in the student body. The faculty is also multi-national; most of the professors have been recruited from medical schools in the United States, Canada, and the U.K.

In addition to an active Dean of Students' office, there are numerous student organizations and a wide range of student support services, including the Department of Educational Services and a Counseling Service, to support the educational programs and student well-being.

General Statement On Admissions Standards From The Admissions Office

The selection of students is made after careful consideration of many aspects: academic ability, emotional and professional maturity, academic achievement, community service, indicators of responsibility and motivation, MCAT scores (when applicable), health professions' experience, and letters of recommendation regarding the applicant's personal qualities, character, motivation, and academic abilities.

Note from the Publisher: Please refer to the section titled "Admission Requirements" on page 3 for a list of specific undergraduate courses required as part of the premedical curriculum for admission.

STUDENT PROFILE
August 1996 & January 1997 Entering Class

In Their Own Words...

Admission Data From The Staff Of St. George's Univ.

ACADEMIC DISTRIBUTIONS		
Grade Point Averages (GPA) of Accepted Students		
Average GPAs	August 1996	January 1997
Overall Undergraduate GPA	3.4	3.3
Science Undergraduate GPA	3.3	3.2
Graduate School GPA	3.5	3.5

AVERAGE MCAT SCORES OF ACCEPTED STUDENTS		
Average MCAT Scores	August 1996	January 1997
Verbal Reasoning	8	8
Physical Sciences	8	9
Biological Sciences	9	9

USMLE I & USMLE II PASS RATES		
	June 1996 USMLE I	August 1996 USMLE II
Overall	81%	67%
First Time Test Takers	88%	50%
U.S. Citizens First Time Test Takers	89%	56%

Note: 94% of the Spring, 1996 St. George's graduates had passed USMLE II prior to graduation.

A recent press release (February, 1997) from the Public Affairs Department of St. George's University School of Medicine is shown below. Please contact Margaret Lambert, Dean of Enrollment Planning or the Admissions Office for further information regarding the content of this press release.

St. George's University
SCHOOL OF MEDICINE
University Centre
Grenada, West Indies

NEWS

For Information
Arthur Massolo
Phone: 516/665-8500
Fax: 516/666-7609

For Immediate Release:

U.S. DEPARTMENT OF EDUCATION
FINDS GRENADA STANDARDS TO ACCREDIT MEDICAL SCHOOL
COMPARABLE TO U.S.

The U.S. Department of Education has officially notified Grenada that the standards by which it accredits the School of Medicine at St. George's University are "comparable to those used to evaluate programs leading to the MD degree in the United States."

Grenada was told Wednesday, February 12, that it was one of four countries in the world that has been so identified. The other countries are Australia, United Kingdom, and Canada. In all, 26 other nations were considered for evaluation.

Prime Minister Keith Mitchell welcomed the news and issued a statement that the "identification of the School of Medicine for its standards of excellence will benefit Grenada and the entire Caribbean region."

In 1994, the U. S. Department of Education established the National Commission for Medical Education and Accreditation. This commission was formed pursuant to the Higher Education Amendment of 1992.

Since then, the NCFMEA has evaluated accreditation standards that apply to foreign medical schools seeking to become, or remain, eligible to participate in the Federal Family Education Loan Program. The commission was charged with determining whether these standards are comparable with those that apply to medical schools in the United States.

The Chancellor of St. George's University, Charles R. Modica, noted that when U.S. Secretary of Education, Richard W. Riley, announced the formation of the National Commission he had stated, "the commission will play a vital role in assuring that federal loans supported by tax-payer dollars only go to foreign medical schools that provide a high quality education to its students." The Chancellor added, "We are proud St. George's has been deemed such an institution." Citing the fact that the University is celebrating its 20th anniversary since it was established in Grenada, he said, "it is gratifying to have the excellent quality of our medical program recognized as such by the U. S. Department of Education by their recent action. Our international faculty has worked hard to achieve this recognition and takes pride in the fact that 88.1% of the students who took Step I of the U. S. Medical Licensing Examination (USMLE) last June passed on the first try."

GRADUATE PROFILE

Runar Sigurdsson, M.D.
Class of '90

Runar Sigurdsson, M.D., a native of Reykjavik, Iceland, gravitated to medicine by way of two careers and a degree in economics.

He started out as a teacher, working for a year in Iceland. Then he worked as a police officer for three years. His contact with people in emergency situations and the doctors who helped them gave him a desire for yet another career change. He began to wonder just how difficult it would be to become a doctor. He would be nearly thirty by the time he began his medical studies, providing he could find a school that would accept him.

St. George's University School of Medicine recognized Runar's desire and his intellectual ability. "To prepare for medical school, I went to the "States" to study pre-med for one year. Once I had completed the courses I needed, I enrolled in St. George's program."

The change from life in Iceland was dramatic. Besides the welcome difference in climate, living conditions were an adjustment for a person who had lived independently and privately. Four roommates shared one room the first semester at St. George's. But Dr. Sigurdsson notes, "We were two Americans, a Nigerian and myself, all very keen on what we were doing. We concentrated on our work and were very supportive of each other."

His work at St. George's took two years, with a fifth semester in St. Vincent, followed by four semesters of clinical studies in England. Dr. Sigurdsson worked for a year in Iceland and then returned to England to take the PLAB exam, which allowed him to undertake an internship in Birmingham and a rotation of family medicine in Canterbury.

"You must be very determined and not expect an easy ride. You need to be prepared for work that requires long hours and for continuing education throughout your career."

When asked what advice he might have for a potential student at St. George's, Dr. Sigurdsson said, "You must be very determined and not expect an easy ride. You need to be prepared for work that requires long hours and for continuing education throughout your career."

During his studies, he met his future wife, Dr. Amanda Scarlett, who is now a family practitioner in England. They live in Herne Bay, a little village outside Canterbury.

Dr. Sigurdsson also noted, "My wife and I both agree that our day goes by very fast. Weeks fly and we are never bored. But when we have had 48 hours on call with very little sleep, we are irritable. Anyone going into medicine must expect good times and bad times and try to keep a balance."

GRADUATE PROFILE

David V. Mlambo, M.D.
Class of '83

David Mlambo, M.D., grew up at Mount Selinda, a Zimbabwe mission run by Americans affliliated with the United Church of Christ. His father was headmaster of both the primary school and the secondary school and his mother was a teacher there. Dr. Mlambo remembers admiring the American doctors at the mission. He watched as people received the help they needed, and he found himself asking, "Why can't I do this?" He decided to pursue medicine as his profession.

When he was ready for college, he traveled to the United States to study biology and chemistry at Western Michigan University. When he began to look for medical schools in the US, he found many doors were closed to foreigners. St. George's University School of Medicine, which was a relatively new school in 1979, was interested in finding dedicated students whose goals were to return to their countries to help alleviate the severe shortages of medical personnel. When Dr. Mlambo was accepted to St. George's, he knew his dream of being a doctor was on its way to becoming a reality. He also knew that there would be hardship. He had married a native Zimbabwean while in the US, but his wife and newborn child would have to stay behind in Michigan. He traveled to Grenada to study and returned to them at the end of each semester.

"You must be dedicated to your chosen career. Prepare to be hard working. You will reap rewards late, so don't look back, always look to the future.

Dr. Mlambo's education at St. George's University School of Medicine has made it possible for him to become a successful doctor. After his graduation in 1983, Dr. Mlambo and his family returned to Zimbabwe. He fulfilled a requirement that called for working in a government institution for five years. He then went on to become the Medical Superintendent of the largest hospital of Zimbabwe: Perirenyatwa Group of Hospitals, the main teaching hospital of the University of Zimbabwe Medical School. "My clinical years at St. George's University School of Medicine were divided between Great Britain and the United States. It was excellent preparation. In particular, going to England gave me insight into the way medicine would be practiced in Zimbabwe."

Now Dr. Mlambo has an office in the center of Harare, the capital city of Zimbabwe. He is the Director of Medical Services for T.A. Holdings, Ltd., the largest wholly Zimbabwean-owned company in the country. He sees employees of the conglomerate of companies and their dependents.

When asked if he has any advice for potential medical students, Dr. Mlambo replied, "You must be dedicated to your chosen career. Prepare to be hard working. You will reap rewards late, so don't look back, always to the future."

▶ **GRENADA 101**

by Jose V. Sumaquial, 3rd year student

While the welcome mat has been rolled out to the student body, seasoned veterans and greenhorns alike, I would like to jump on the welcoming bandwagon and extend my salutations to one and all. While most of the upper classmen have expectations of the school and the island, I'd like to give the first term students a crash course in adjusting to your newfound home and lifestyle. Let me start with a scenario not unfamiliar to past students.

You've had a long, rigorous trip with multiple layovers at various airports to reach your final destination: Port Salines Airport. Reality slams you in the face as you step off the stale, air-conditioned plane and are engulfed by the heat and humidity. You sigh at the long lines at the Port of Entry booths, luggage carousels, and finally Customs. You feel like a lost sheep as a handful of orientation staffers direct you to the Grand Anse or True Blue line. Upon depositing your precious luggage in one of the many St. George's flatbed trucks, you and your comrades are now herded into buses, "packed like lemmings into shiny metal boxes." Present first-termers will appreciate the taxi service provided by the school. As you proceed through the pothole-ridden streets on to your destination to either campus, you notice the lush vegetation, the rather aggressive local driving habits, and the HEAT. As you pull into the Grand Anse campus, you notice the Gross Anatomy Department, the Simon Bolivar Clinic and the Grand Anse Dorms. Overwhelmed by everything, you keep thinking to yourself, " What the hell am I getting myself into?"

It's a fact that every student on this island has had to ask himself or herself that same question at one time or another. But I'm here to tell you that things are great in Grenada; you simply need to open your eyes and embrace the campus and the Grenadine lifestyle for what it is. The key here is not to expect this country to be the United States, because it's not! We are in Grenada, a beautiful country with warm and friendly citizens. So here are a few tips to get you acclimated to the island.

ATTITUDE – First and foremost, the attitude you carry with you will directly affect your stay in Grenada. I mentioned earlier to keep an open mind. This will help you in your adjustment to the slower, laid-back lifestyle of the island. Since most of us have been spoiled with the conveniences and modern amenities of the U.S., you'll soon learn to appreciate little privileges that we at home consider "god-given rights", like air conditioning and a good supply of hot water. Also, contrary to what you may think right now, you all should be proud to be here. It is not an easy feat to receive an acceptance here.

(I am sure this fact has been or will be conveyed to you during orientation.)

ACTIVITIES – As first term students experiencing culture shock, the best way to cope with your new home is to approach your stay here as a two year extended vacation. Therefore, take the time to see the island. The best means of doing that is to take advantage of the school sponsored tours held before orientation of each first term class. If you miss them, try taking one the following term. The island is very beautiful, offering rain forests, white sand beaches, waterfalls and two seas (the Caribbean blue waters to the west and the darker waters of the Atlantic to the east). Take some time out on a Saturday morning to visit the city of St. George and the farmers market. There is a movie theater that shows pseudo-current movies as well as a plethora of international films, including my favorite, dubbed Kung Fu movies. As for clubs, most students frequent the Boat Yard on Fridays and Saturdays as well as Cot Bam (adjacent to the G.A. Campus) for a more social atmosphere. Bolero seems to be a new fad .

> *"...The island is very beautiful, offering rain forests, white sand beaches, waterfalls..."*

MONEY – There are several banks near the Grand Anse Campus in which most students keep their money, two of which have ATM machines for added convenience. You can have money wired have travelers checks and money orders cashed, or as take out cash advances on your credit card. If you take out cash advances, consider AMEX or Discover card first, for the lack of interest rate and lower fees, respectively. The ATM machine also allows the payment of phone and electric bills. Make sure before you go to cash a money order that the check is co-signed by the school in the Accounting/ Procurement Department. The current rate of exchange is about $2.67 E.C. per $1 U.S.

MAIL – If you do not already know, the school mail room is located on the Grand Anse Campus across from the Copy Center (near the bus stop). Ashton and Eric are there to distribute mail and sell some supplemental books, laundry tokens (at $1 E.C. each) and other things. Mail can also be deposited at the library desk at True Blue. There are fax machines in the library, student center and chancellory. Faxes or mail to Medical School Services can be sent with the help of Dawn Buckmire in the Housing/Financial Aid office.

TRANSPORTATION – A first termer's best friend is the bus schedule which you can pick up at the Mailroom. It is especially helpful in time management, as you will find out soon enough. Some students do purchase automobiles (usually used). However, you must obtain a local driver's license to drive in Grenada. There are temporary licenses, which last for three months, available at the traffic department at the Police station at the cost of $30 E.C. There is also a year-long license available for $60 E.C. Besides the St. George's school bus, students often take "reggae" buses (attributed to the music played in them) to various parts of the island. Usually for the price of $1 E.C., these buses will take you to almost anywhere on the island.

FOOD – The most convenient places to get food are on campus, i.e. Green Jeans and the "ladies" on Grand Anse, and the Sugar Shack on the True Blue Campus. The "ladies" at Grand Anse, local women who prepare food for students, offer reasonably priced meals (usually about $20E.C. for a huge dinner) or a meal plan can be arranged with them. There are also a variety of nearby restaurants which students frequent, including Jade Garden (offering Chinese Food), Rick's Cafe (a pizzeria and ice cream shop) and the Boulangerie, all having very reasonable prices. To store your leftovers and other perishable items, refrigerator rentals can be obtained from Riley's (440-8268) and other local businesses. They are usually on campus during the beginning of each term distributing refrigerators to those living in the dorms. The average cost of refrigerator rental per semester is $140 U.S.

Also, expect a little time for your stomach to adjust to the water. Most students drink bottled water. It is also a good idea to keep some bottled water with you to prevent dehydration. Plus, the faculty allows no food or drink of any sort, except for water, in the new lecture hall.

SHOPPING – Every Saturday morning, there is a farmers market in the town of St. George. Groceries can be bought at Food Fair , "D" Green Grocer (both located near campus), and Foodland. Courts, Hubbards, True Value/Huggins and Ace Hardware carry many household items from Tupperware and dishes to transformers. Hubbards and Foodland do offer a 5% discount to medical students.

STUDYING –This is the real reason we are all here. However, there is more than ample time to do other activities. It is really easy to burn out quickly, especially in a place so far from home. So take some time out for yourself. A good night's rest is also important. If you feel the need to take part in other activities on campus addressing some of the concerns of the campus and the island, there are opportunities in student government as well as involvement in AMSA. Some of these activities can help you realize the true meaning of your stay here: to become a physician. For instance, the two health fairs sponsored by AMSA give you opportunities to come in direct contact with patients. Also, AMSA, the EM Club and others, sponsor clinic visits and lectures of medical interest.

"Also, expect a little time for your stomach to adjust to the water. Most students drink bottled water. It is also a good idea to keep some bottled water with you to prevent dehydration."

So in closing, I would just like to say that you have been given the opportunity for a very unique medical education. I suggest that you take advantage of the assets the school and the island have to offer. You will become better people and certainly better doctors. Good Luck!

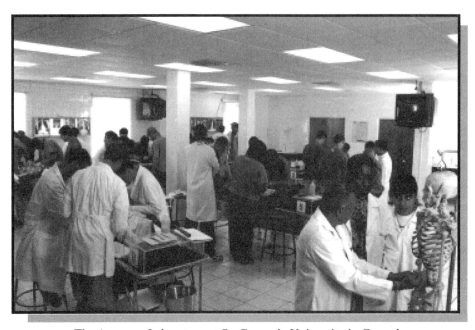

The Anatomy Laboratory at St. George's University in Grenada

The Best of the Bunch

Dominica
West Indies

The Country Fact Box
DOMINICA

- *Capital:* Roseau
- *Government:* Parliamentary Democracy
- *Head of Government:* Prime Minister
- *Population:* 83,000
- *Primary Languages:* English & French
  patois
- *Monetary Unit:* East Caribbean Dollar

Ross University
School of Medicine

Portsmouth

Ross University
School of Medicine

Office of Admissions • International Education Admissions
460 West 34th Street (12th Floor) • New York • NY 10001
Phone: New York (212) 279-5500 • California (818) 248-0812
Florida (305) 899-8151 • Michigan (810) 539-9255
Fax: (212) 629-3147
Email: admissions@rossmed.edu • Internet: http://www.rossmed.edu

Ross University School of Medicine was founded by Dr. Robert Ross in 1978. At the beginning, Ross University was known as the University of Dominica. The first class entered the University in April, 1979. Since then more than 2,000 students have graduated and earned their M.D. degree from Ross University. According to the University, graduates have gone on to practice medicine in a wide variety of specialties including transplant nephrology, neonatalogy, infectious diseases, plastic surgery, and hematology/oncology. In addition, the University adds that "a significant number of alumni have gone on to become chief residents and associate clinical professors at U.S. medical schools..." The student body is both multi-national and multi-ethnic at Ross University. However, a large number of students hail from the U.S. Additionally, the faculty of the medical school is represented by professors from around the world.

Ross University School of Medicine is chartered by the government of Dominica. The University is also recognized in the World Health Organization's *World Directory of Medical Schools*. Students enrolled at Ross University complete the basic sciences curriculum on-campus on the island of Dominica, while clinical rotations are completed in Dominica, the United Kingdom, and the U.S. Currently, the University is exploring the possibility of developing clinical programs in Canada.

Location

▶ Dominica, The Caribbean Basin

The basic sciences campus of Ross University is located in Portsmouth, Dominica. Portsmouth lies on the northern end of the island of Dominica.

Dominica was discovered by Columbus in 1493. Until 1978, the island remained a British colony. The island of Dominica is twenty-nine miles long and sixteen miles wide. It receives 40 inches to 300 inches of rain annually. Because of heavy rainfall, Dominica is laced with lush foliage that drapes the island's many waterfalls and volcanic peaks. The abundance of scenic sights have earned Dominica the nickname of "Nature Island of the Caribbean." The island is also known for having the best snorkling and scuba spots in the entire Caribbean region.

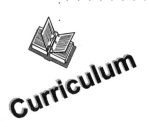

► **The Medical Program**

The M.D. program at Ross University is designed to be completed in four calender years. The first academic year is divided into three semesters while the second academic year consists of two semesters.

Students spent the first two calender years on the island of Dominica. During this period, students matriculate in the basic sciences program which concentrates on the traditional medical science disciplines. Through a combination of class lectures, small-group discussions, computer-assisted instructions and laboratory sessions, the basics of fundamental sciences are conveyed to students. Some of the subjects covered during basic sciences include Gross Anatomy, Physiology, Histology, Medical Cell Biology, Biochemistry, and Neuroscience.

The next two years of the program are clinically oriented during which students spend most of their time working in university affiliated hospitals. During the first 48 of the 75 weeks, students enter clinical rotations in departments of medicine, surgery, obstetrics/gynecology (OB/GYN), family medicine, psychiatry and pediatrics. The remaining 27 weeks are set aside for elective rotations. Students may choose to enroll in various medical subspecialties during this period. All clinical rotations are completed in Ross University's affliated hospitals in the Caribbean, the United Kingdom and the U.S. *(the list of affliated hospitals is published below)*.

 ► **The Official Clinical Affiliation List**

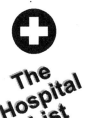

United States
Brooklyn Hospital, Brooklyn, NY
Jamaica Hospital, Queens, NY
Maryland General Hospital, Baltimore, MD
Kern County Hospital, Bakersfield, CA
Danbury Hospital, Danbury, CT
St. Mary's Hospital, Waterbury, CT
Jackson Park Hospital, Chicago, IL

In addition to these hospitals, the University has other affiliated clinical sites in Arizona, California, Connecticut, Illinois, Maryland, Massachusetts, Missouri and Ohio.

Students at Ross University also complete their clinical clerkships at hospitals located in the Caribbean and the United Kingdom.

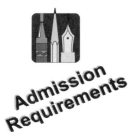

Minimum Admission Requirements

The minimum admission requirements for applicants from North America (the United States and Canada) are as follows:

- A bachelor's degree from an accredited university or college prior to matriculation into the University.
- Completion of premedical curriculum that includes the following courses:
    1. General biology with laboratory – one year (two semesters)
    2. Inorganic chemistry with laboratory – one year (two semesters)
    3. Organic chemistry with laboratory – one year (two semesters)
    4. Physics with laboratory – one year (two semesters)
    5. Mathematics (preferably Calculus) – one semester
    6. English – one year (two semesters)
- OPTIONAL: Medical College Admission Test (MCAT) score

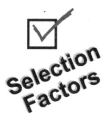

Selection Factors

According to the official University brochure, the selection of a student "… is considered on the basis of his or her academic record, letters of recommendation, and the student's record of involvement in college and community activities…" It is important to note that the admissions committee did not rank the various selection factors in any order of importance. The Admissions Committee also considers applicants' motivation for the study of medicine in its decision making process.

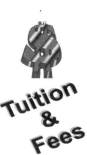

Tuition & Fees

Term:	Basic Sciences Semesters 1,2, and 3 (Year #1 & #2)		
Campus:	Portsmouth, Dominica		
Pre-clinical	$6790 per term(15-17 credits/semester) $453 per cerdit (<15 credits)		
Fees	Matriculation: $250	Library Fee: $60/semester	Printed Materials Fee: $250
Term	Clinical Years 1 & 2		
Clinicals	$7190 per semester		
Other Costs	Textbooks and clinical clothing purchase		
Evacuation Insurance	$ 65 per calender year (if bought through Ross)		
Malpractice Fee	$ 600 per calender year		
Graduation Fee	$ 500		

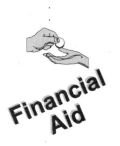

Financial Aid

Most students attending medical school at Ross University receive some form of financial aid. The Office of Student Financial Planning assists students with financial planning and budgeting. The vast majority of the financial aid packages received by students are in the form of loans. Ross University's students are eligible for both governmental and private loans in the United States and Canada. No information was available regarding University merit or need based scholarships.

- *Government Loan Programs (USA):*
    1. The Subsidized Federal Stafford program – $8,500 per year
    2. The Unsubsidized Federal Stafford program – $10,000 per year
    3. The Canada Student Loan Program *(Canadian citizens only)*

- *Private Educational Loan Programs:*
    1. International Health Education Loan Program

- *Veterans' Benefits:*
    1. Eligible U.S. veterans may use benefits available through the VA towards their educational costs.

Student Life

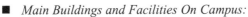

The University conducts its basic medical sciences curriculum at the main campus located in Portsmouth, in the northern portion of Dominica. It is approximately one hour away from the Dominican capital city of Roseau.

- *Main Buildings and Facilities On Campus:*
    1. Main Academic Building (includes classrooms and laboratory)
    2. Administration Building (includes a 300-seat auditorium)
    3. Learning Resources Center
    4. 250-seat Auditorium classroom building
    5. Cafeteria Building
    6. Weight room, tennis and basketball courts
    7. Day Care Center

- *Housing On Campus:*
  There are no university owned on-campus dormitories for students. However, Ross's housing coordinators help students find decent accommodations in the Portsmouth area. The majority of the students live within the close proximity of the Basic Sciences campus.
  Students are advised by the University to contact the Housing Director and arrange for suitable accommodations prior to their departure from the U.S.

- *Student Organizations*
  1. Student Government Association
  2. American Medical Student Association (AMSA) chapter
  3. Organized Religious Services – Christian, Hindu, Jewish, Muslim, and Buddhist

- *Life Outside The Campus*
  The warm climate of Dominica dictates the lifestyle of the people on the island. Dominica offers ample opportunities for outdoor activities. Students can engage in numerous aquatic activities including swimming, wind-surfing, diving and snorkeling in the blue waters of the Caribbean Sea.

  Dominica is a typical Caribbean island full of "photo ops". No wonder the island is known as the "Nature Island of the Caribbean". Nature lovers will find the lush tropical vegetation ideal for photography. In addition, Dominica is home to some of the most magnificient beaches in the world. Students take full advantage off the numerous natural attarctions by exploring them during their free time. Majestic waterfalls, tranquil pools, and Valley of Desolation and Boiling Lake are few of the natural wonders that dot the island of Dominica. Beautiful natural trails await those of you who enjoy hiking and sightseeing.

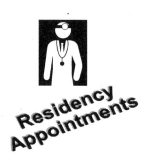

Residency Appointments

Recent Residency Appointments

The following list is a sample of various residency programs entered by graduating members of the Classes of 1990-95:

Internal Medicine
Danbury Hospital, CT
St. Luke's Hospital, MO
Maricopa Medical Center, AZ
Medical College of Virginia, VA
Kern Medical Center, CA
St. John's Hospital, MI
Drew Medical Center, CA
McNeal hospital, IL

Yale Primary Care, CT
Univ of Louisville, KY
West Suburban Hospital Center, IL
Roger Williams Hospital, RI
UMDNJ Hospital, NJ
Sacred Heart Hospital, WA
Hackensack Medical Center, NJ
Christ Hospital & Medical Center, IL
Hahnemann University Hospital, PA

Pediatrics
University of Texas Medical Cntr, TX
Michigan State University, MI

Emergency Medicine & Anesthesiology
Medical College of Wisconsin, WI
Christ Hospital, IL
Phramonkutlao Hospital, Thailand
Medical Center of Georgia, GA

General Surgery & Specialty Surgery
Mit. Sinai Medical Center, FL
Lincoln Hospital, Bronx, NY
St. Agnes Hospital, MD
Moffit Hospital, San Francisco, CA
Hahnemann Hospital, PA
Drew Medical Center, CA
St. Raphael's Hospital, CT
Union Memorial Hospital, MD
West Suburban Hospital. IL

Psychiatry, Opthalmology & Medicine	Family Practice & OB/GYN
Robert Wood Johnson Med Cntr, NJ	Methodist Medical Center, IL
Univ of South Carolina, SC	Robert Wood Johnson Med Cntr, NJ
Stamford Hospital, CT	University of Buffalo, NY
	Medical College of Virginia, VA
	St. John's Hospital, MI
	Bon Secours Hospital, MI
	St. Francis Hospital, KS
	Carbondale Memorial Hospital, IL
	Richland Memorial Hospital, SC
	Wayne State University. MI
	Still Regional Hospital, MO
	Prince George's Hospital, MD
	Howard University Hospital, Washington, DC

The Daily Survival Guide

Attending medical school classes is only a part of your life in Dominica. The daily survival guide below lists some of the useful information you need to know about life in Dominica.

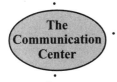

The Communication Center

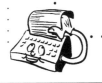

Phone Calls Home
USA Direct Lines – Dial "1" followed by the rest of the telephone number including the area code.

Postal Service
Regular air-mails from Dominica to the US require .90 EC cents and postcards require .55 EC cents. UPS service is available from Dominica.

Fax Service
Ross's Student Government Copy provides FAX services to students. Students are charged a minimal fee for outbound faxes.

Food and Supermarkets
American style food is available in the two University-owned cafeterias. In the central open market, local vendors sell fresh fruits and vegetables. The typical Dominican diet includes chicken, fish and lots of vegetables and fruits.

Electricity Supply Check
Dominica's electrical supply is 220 volts and 50 hertz.

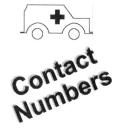

Contact Numbers

IN CASE OF EMERGENCY

University Chancellory
Ross University, Dominica
Phone#: (809)445-5355
Fax#: (809)445-5383

Dean of Students Office (Dominica)
Dr. John Corbett, Dean
Phone#: (809)445-3104

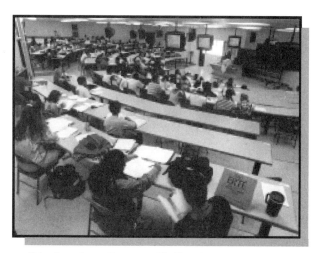

Biochemistry Lecture Hall at Ross's campus
in Dominica

1996 General Admissions Data			
Entering Class	**Applications Received**	**Accepted Applicants**	**New Entrants**
January 1996	541	274	192
May 1996	456	268	164
September 1996	976	438	195

STUDENT PROFILE
January 1997 Entering Class

ACADEMIC DISTRIBUTIONS	
Grade Point Averages (GPA) of Accepted Students	
Cumulative Class GPA (average)	3.12
Cumulative Prerequisite GPA	3.13
Cumulative Advanced Biology GPA	3.25
Cumulative Graduate School GPA	3.31
GPA Cohort Percentages	
GPA above 3.5	15.80%
GPA between 3.0 & 3.5	50.45%
GPA between 2.75 & 3.0	21.00%
GPA below 2.75	12.40%

DISTRIBUTION OF TYPES OF DEGREES	
Undergraduate	
BA	28%
BS	68%
Other	3.5%
Graduate	
MS, MPH, DC, PhD & MBA	22 students

In Their Own Words...

Comments From The Staff Of Ross University

GENDER, AGE, AND ETHNIC DISTRIBUTIONS

Gender	Men: 66.30% Women: 33.70%

Age Cohorts

Between 20 & 25 years of age	49%
Between 25 & 30 years of age	27.80%
Between 30 & 35 years of age	13%
Between 35 & 40 years of age	4.80%
Between 40 & 45 years of age	3.40%
Between 45 & 50 years of age	1.40%

Ethnic Origins

White	35.40%
Indian/Pakistani	25%
Middle Eastern	14.90%
Asian (China, Korea, etc.)	14%
African American	7.60%
Hispanic	3%

Undergraduate Universities Attended by Students of January 1997 Entering Class

Adelphi University	Long Island Univ.	Temple University
Boston University	Loyola University	Trenton State College
Brigham Young Univ.	Montclair State Univ.	Tufts University
California State Univ.	NYU	Tulane University
CUNY	Northwestern Univ.	US Naval Academy
Cleveland State Univ.	Ohio State Univ.	US Military Academy
Columbia University	Pace University	USC
Cooper Union	Penn State University	Univ. of California
Cornell University	RIT	Univ. of Florida
Dartmouth College	Rutgers University	University of Illinois
Florida State Univ.	San Diego State	University of Maryland
Fordham University	San Francisco State	University of Michigan
Hahnemann University	Sonoma State Univ.	Univ. of Pennsylvania
Hunter College	SUNY	University of Rochester
Johns Hopkins Univ.	Syracuse University	University of Texas

What Medical Students At Ross Said

How hard is medical school?
We'd be lying if we said it was easy. But, it is not impossible. There are doctors everywhere. Studying has to be done every night. The amount of the material is incredible, yet interesting. It will be intimidating at first. Don't get discouraged – just keep working at it and you'll be pleased with the results.

Don't you have to be at the top of your class to succeed?
There is an old saying that says "The Big P=MD" (P meaning Pass); this is true to a certain extent. We are NOT saying just squeek by, but try your best. If you pass and know enough to do well on the Boards, you'll be fine. The better you do on the boards, the more opportunities and doors will open for you in the clinical portion of the program. This is also true for residency programs.

What is the campus like?
The campus has lots of mango, coconut and banana trees around it, which is great for snacks. The classrooms are equipped with TV monitors that project supplemental material during lectures to ensure that everyone can read what is being discussed. We also have a stereo sound system to make sure that no one misunderstands what is being said. The library is quite large and contains a computer lab with the latest medical education software. It also has an extensive selection of periodicals and resource materials. The campus is air conditioned almost to the point of freezing, but stepping outside to warm up usually cures this. Students have individual lockers and can be seen congregating around them in some type of heated discussion.

What is living on Dominica really like?
It takes some getting used to. But it has a charm of its own. You will get frustrated at times, but after awhile you get used to it. It is a wonderful experience that really teaches you about humility. The living conditions are adequate. Do not be shocked by the differences. Medical school is for studying and allows little time for anything else. Dominica offers natural distractions to calm your nerves when you need it, and waves to sing you to sleep after a hard day. The mosquitoes and insects are manageable. Living in Dominica is nothing to be afraid of and can be quite enjoyable if you let it.

What do you do for fun?
After exams, some students drink a few beers and dance to trendy Dominican songs at Coconuts. Also, there are social events planned by the SGA, such as an island tour, numerous parties, lunches and dinners, special holiday events, a talent show, sports competitions and weekly movies at the school or in Portsmouth. In addition, there is a plethora of water sports and outdoor activities.

In Their Own Words...

Comments From Current Medical Students at Ross University

Do the professors give out handouts before class and do they teach adequately?
Most professors distribute handouts before class and rarely do they not give some type of supplemental material. On the whole, our professors are wonderful; they know the students on a personal, first-name basis and care about their students' well being. Some professors are better than others, but that is true of any school.

Is there a big problem with crime?
There have been very few incidents of serious crime, but this is a very poor island and petty theft can be a problem. The police are excellent in catching and reprimanding criminals and this is a big deterrent. In addition, Ross University has 24-hour security with trained, uniformed personnel. They patrol the school and student housing to help ensure the safety of the students.

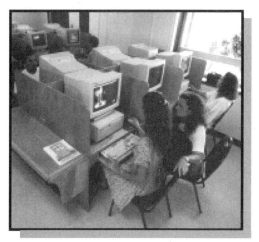

The Learning Resource Laboratory
at Ross University's Portsmouth
campus in Dominica

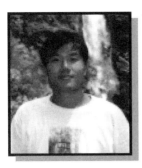

MIKE LIU
Second year medical student at Ross University

- M.P.H. – Loma Linda University, Loma Linda, CA
  Major: Environmental Health
- B.A. – University of California, Berkeley, CA
  Major: Molecular and Cell Biology

In his own words:

Meet A Ross Medical Student

Looking back at my first year and a half at Ross University, I must say the greatest adjustment lies in adapting to the living conditions of Dominica. The rude welcome I received from Hurricane Luis and Hurricane Marilyn in 1995, set the stage for an enduring journey. For example, there are no-self service laundries. I have to hire a local woman to wash my clothes, and the turnaround time may be two or three days depending on the weather. "Supermarkets," as we know them in the United States can be found only in the capital city of Roseau, which is an hour away from Portsmouth (the city where the Ross campus is located). Students usually buy their groceries from smaller stores around the school. Although there are a couple of nearby vegetable and fruit stands, the outdoor Saturday morning market is the best source of quality vegetables and fruits. While Dominica is an island nation surrounded by oceans on all sides, the availability of fresh fish is limited. Most of the prepared meals consist of chicken and rice. Yes, the Dominican standard of living differs vastly from American living standards. At times, the disparity between the two can be overwhelming. In sharing my thoughts, however, I hope not to discourage anyone who dreams of becoming a doctor. Instead, I wish to convey the message that the hardship of attending medical school abroad can be overcome if you are prepared to handle an adventure of a lifetime.

- **THE STATE OF THE CLASSROOMS AND OTHER FACILITIES**

Where does the majority of the lectures take place?
Mostly in lecture halls, but sometimes in classrooms.

What are the capacities of most classrooms and lecture halls?
Largest classroom – 150 seats
Largest lecture hall – 200 seats

Is the primary lecture hall air-conditioned, well lit and comfortable?
Generally, the lecture halls are air-conditioned, well lit and comfortable.

Are scientific journals available at the school?
Most journals are available in the library.

Are laboratories large, well equipped and well lit?
The labs are adequate. A new anatomy lab is under construction.
The histology/pathology lab is sufficient.

What is the capacity of the anatomy laboratory?
100 students.

Is the anatomy laboratory well ventillated and air-conditioned?
The Anatomy lab is air-conditioned. New lab is under construction.

How many students are assigned to each cadaver during anatomy dissection sessions?
10 to 15 students.

What is the condition of the laboratory equipment? Has it been upgraded to match the latest products found on the market? Is there enough equipment such as microscopes? Does your school provide you with latex gloves?
The students need to provide their own gloves for dissection and their own microscopes for histology and pathology labs.

> *"The students need to provide their own gloves for dissection and their own microscopes for histology and pathology labs."*

Are dining facilities adequate? Briefly, describe the availability of food on-campus.
There are two dining facilities on campus: Seaside Cafeteria and Cafe Jolle. In addition, various independent vendors also sell food at the gate. In general, food is adequate, but the variety can be improved.

Are student recreational facilities adequate? Briefly, describe the various recreational facilities on-campus.
There are two tennis courts, one basketball court, one volleyball court, and a weight room on-campus. Weekly aerobic classes are also conducted on-campus.

On a scale of 1 to 10, rate your overall satisfaction with your school's current classrooms and other facilities – 1 (least satisfied) and 10 (most satisfied).
7

On a scale of 1 to 10, rate your overall satisfaction with your school's current laboratory facilities – 1 (least satisfied) and 10 (most satisfied).
5

■ **THE STATE OF THE ACADEMICS**

How accessible are the professors?
Overall, the professors are very accessible. Most can be reached for
questions and answers.

Is the library adequate?
In general, the library serves its purpose. Most journals are available
there. Seating capacity can be improved. The library is open 24
hours a day prior to major examinations.

Is there an on-campus computer facility? If so, how many computer
terminals and printers are available for student use?
Yes, there is an on-campus computer room. Approximately 30
computers and 6 printers are available for student use.

Do students have access to on-line databases such as the Medline?
Yes

Do students have access to the Internet and have e-mail accounts?
Yes

What types of other academic related services are available to
students (i.e.: tutoring, copying service, note translation service, etc.)
Counseling is available.

On a scale of 1 to 10, rate your overall satisfaction with your
***school's academics** – 1 (least satisfied) and 10 (most satiesfied).*
5

> *"In general, the*
> *library serves its*
> *purpose. Most*
> *journals are*
> *available there."*

■ **THE STATE OF THE STUDENT BODY & COMMUNITY**

How diverse is the student body? What are the most popular home
states of students from the United States?
The student body is diverse both geographically and ethnically. The
most popular home states are New York, New Jersey, Florida,
California and Illinois.

Do students cooperate amongst each other when it comes to sharing
notes, and old test questions? Are most students "cut-throat" in
nature?
In general, students are cooperative. Usually, transcribed notes and
old examinations can be obtained.

In general, are students happy to be at Ross University or are they
disappointed about their experience of attending medical school
abroad?
Most students attend Ross as a last resort. We are satisfied in
knowing that we are getting a medical education.

Are most students homesick or have they managed to acclimate themselves to the surrounding community in Dominica?
Most students are homesick and are eager to return home to the U.S.

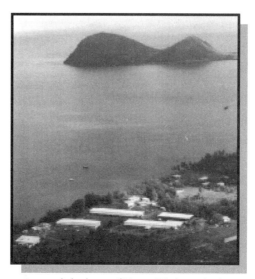

An aerial view of Ross University's
campus at Portsmouth, Dominica

The Best of the Bunch

Tel Aviv

Israel

> **The Country Fact Box**
> **ISRAEL**
>
> - *Capital:* Jerusalem
> - *Government:* Republic
> - *Head of Government:* Prime Minister
> - *Population:* approx. 6,000,000
> - *Primary Languages:* Hebrew and Arabic
> - *Monetary Unit:* Sheqel

Tel Aviv University
Sackler School of Medicine
Tel Aviv

Sackler School of Medicine
New York State–American Program

Office of Admissions
17 East 62nd Street • New York • NY 10021
Phone: 212-688-8811
Fax: 212-223-0368
Internet: http://www.tau.ac.il/~ori/body.html

Tel Aviv University's School of Medicine was established in 1964. In 1972, the school was renamed the Sackler Faculty of Medicine. Currently, it is comprised of Schools of Medicine, Dental Medicine, Continuing Medical Education, and Health Professions.

The Sackler School of Medicine offers programs leading to the M.D. degrees, as well as to M.Sc. (Masters) and Ph.D. degrees. According to the school, more than 600 Israeli students are enrolled in the M.D. program. In addition to the Israeli students, approximately 280 students are also enrolled in Sackler's New York State–American Program. The American Program is designed specifically for students hailing from the United States. The program was established in 1976. The entire program is in English and the curriculum is modeled after those of US medical schools. Currently, the New York State–American Program is accredited by the Regents of the University of the State of New York and the State of Israel.

The American student body at Sackler is mostly from New York, New Jersey and a few other states. The student body is not as diverse as student bodies in comparable schools. The Sackler faculty is widely recognized for the high quality of its research, which has produced significant medical discoveries. According to Sackler's official brochure "…many have been invited to participate in projects with the National Institutes of Health and other prestigious American research organizations, as well as with prominent institutes and universities throughout the world."

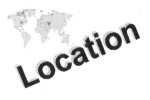

Location

Tel Aviv, Israel

The basic sciences buildings are located on a 170-acre campus in the Tel Aviv suburb of Ramat Aviv. Tel Aviv is a large cosmopolitan city of approximately 1.5 million people. The city is rich with history and culture. The mix of European and Middle Eastern cultures help to generate the unique lifestyle of the city. Unfortunately, the constant threat of terroristic violence is a large part of life in Tel Aviv.

The country of Israel is located in the Middle East bordered by Egypt, Syria and Jordan. Israel is a country full of historical, archaeological and natural treasures. Although conflict is a significant part of life in Israel, the western-style lifestyle makes for quite comfortable living.

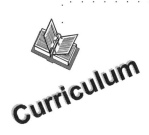

Curriculum

The Medical Program

The New York State-American medical curriculum at Sackler School of Medicine is four years long. The curriculum is divided into two traditional parts – preclinical and clinical.

During the first two years of the program, basic sciences are taught through lectures, laboratory sessions, small group discussions and individual studies. Preclinical science courses include Anatomy, Neuropharmacology, Behavioral Sciences, Biochemistry, Cellular Physiology, Immunology, General Pathology, Microbiology and more. In addition, students are introduced to clinical medicine through the physician advisor and clinical correlation programs. Part of the basic sciences education involves analysis of cases presented by senior physicians.

The third and fourth years are dedicated to clinical training. The practice of clinical medicine begins in the hospital with physical diagnosis, near the end of the second year. Students are involved in all aspects of patient care during their clinical training. The major required clerkships in internal medicine, pediatrics, surgery, obstetrics and gynecology, and psychiatry are taken during the third year. In the fourth year, students complete various elective rotations to gain further insight into the practice of medicine.

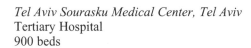

The Official Clinical Affiliation List

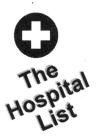

The Hospital List

Sackler School of Medicine Affiliated Hospitals

Tel Aviv Sourasku Medical Center, Tel Aviv
Tertiary Hospital
900 beds

Chaim Sheba Medical Center, Tel Aviv
Tertiary Hospital
1,200 beds

Assaf Harofe Hospital, Rehovot/Ramla Area
Regional Hospital
650 beds

Beilinson Medical Center, Petah Tikva
Tertiary Hospital
1,200 beds

Sapir Medical Center, Kfar Sava
Regional Hospital
590 beds

Golda Meir Medical Center, Petah Tikva
Regional Hospital
384 beds

Edith Wolfson Hospital, Tel Aviv
Regional Hospital
620 beds

Children's Medical Center of Israel, Ra'anana
Tertiary Pediatric Hospital
224 beds

Psychiatric Hospitals – Yehudah Abarbanel, Be'er Ya'akov, Gehah, Nes Ziona & Shalvata Psychiatric Hospitals and the Franz Brill Community Mental Health Center
Tel Aviv area

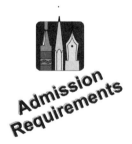

► **Minimum Admission Requirements**

The minimum admission requirements for applicants from the United States are as follows:

- A bachelor's degree from an accredited university or college prior to matriculation into the University.
- Completion of premedical curriculum that includes the following courses:
    1. General biology with laboratory – one year (two semesters)
    2. Inorganic chemistry with laboratory – one year (two semesters)
    3. Organic chemistry with laboratory – one year (two semesters)
    4. Physics with laboratory – one year (two semesters)
    5. English – one year (two semesters)
- Medical College Admission Test (MCAT) score
- Be a citizen or permanent resident of the United States

► **Selection Factors**

According to the official University brochure, the selection of students is based on the following criteria "…in addition to demonstrated academic excellence as reflected by a student's grades and MCAT scores, the Committee carefully evaluates personal qualities such as maturity, integrity, leadership, compassion, empathy and judgment. Sackler prefers service-oriented students who have sincere and realistic motivations for pursuing a career in medicine…". It is important to note that the admissions committee did not rank the various selection factors in any order of importance.

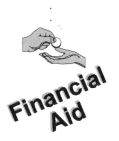

Financial Aid

Attending Sacker can be an expensive proposition for many students. The School recognizes the hardship and employs a Financial Aid Coordinator in the New York office to advise students on matters related to financial aid.

- *Government Loan Programs (USA):*
  1. The Subsidized Federal Stafford program – $8,500 per year
  2. The Unsubsidized Federal Stafford program – $10,000 per year

- *Private Educational Loan Programs:*
  Information not supplied by the school.

- *Institutional Aid Programs (US Students only):*
  Information not supplied by the school.

The Sackler School of Medicine also provides information on bank loan programs to accepted students.

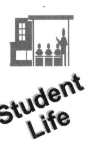

Student Life

Sackler's main campus is located in Tel Aviv. More than 40 modern buildings on the main campus provide teaching, research, residential and recreational facilities to more than 30,000 students. The Sackler School of Medicine is part of the campus and is situated within the premises of a modern 10-story building.

- *Main Buildings & Institutes On Campus:*
  1. Sackler School of Medicine Building
  2. Henry & Grete Abrahams Library of Life Sciences & Medicine
  3. Glasberg Animal Tower
  4. Institute for Human Ecology & Environmental Medicine
  5. The Occupational Health Institute
  6. The Diaspora Museum
  7. Sports facilities including an Olympic-sized pool

- *Life In And Out Of The Campus*
The social, recreational and cultural attributes of Sackler's local and national environment are rich and varied. Israel is a democratic, mostly western-style country. English is the second language of the country. Students can watch English-language news broadcasts on TV and read English newspapers in Tel Aviv.

The campus has a broad range of sports facilities for student use. In addition, activities such as film, theater productions, and concerts are quite high on campus. The temperate climate is ideal for various on-campus outdoor activities.

Tel Aviv is a cosmopolitan city teeming with theaters, concert halls, museums, restaurants, pubs, nightclubs and places of worship. Students can walk to the Mediterranean for swimming, windsurfing and sailing. A large park near the campus is also ideal for walks and picnics. Like any big city, Tel Aviv offers all the amenities associated with large cities.

On occasion, students have the opportunity to venture out of Tel Aviv and explore the rich history of Israel. From Galilee to the Negev Desert to the venerable Jerusalem, students have an unique opportunity to see and experience Israel's varied past and present.

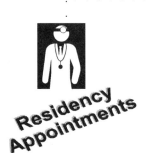

Residency Appointments

▶ Recent Residency Appointments

The following list is a sample of various residency and fellowship programs entered by Sackler students:

Albert Einstein College of Medicine, Bronx, NY	Bridgeport Hospital, Bridgeport, CT
Albany Medical Center, Albany, NY	Brookdale Hospital Center, Brooklyn, NY
Baystate Medical Center, Springfield, MA	Buffalo General Hospital, Buffalo, NY
Beth Israel Medical Center, NY, NY	Case Western Reserve University Hospital, Cleveland, OH
Booth Memorial Hospital, Queens, NY	Children's Memorial Hospital, Chicago, IL
Boston V.A. Medical Center, Boston, MA	Cleveland Clinic, Cleveland, OH
Columbia Presbyterian Medical Center, New York, NY	Hospital for Joint Diseases, NY, NY
The Cornell Hospitals–New York Hospital, New York, NY	Jackson Memorial Hospital, Miami, FL
Danbury Hospital, Danbury, CT	John Hopkins University Children's Medical Center, Baltimore, MD
Denver General Hospital, Denver, CO	Kaiser Permanente Medical Center, Oakland, CA
Duke University Medical Center, Durham, NC	Lenox Hill Hospital, New York, NY
Emory University, Atlanta, GA	Maimonides Medical Center, Brooklyn, NY
Genessee Memorial Hospital, Batavia, NY	Memorial Sloan Kettering Cancer Center, NY, NY
George Washington University Medical Center, Washington, DC	New England Medical Center, Boston, MA
Georgetown Hospital, Washington, DC	University of Pennsylvania, Philadelphia, PA
Greenwich Hospital, Greenwich, CT	Temple University, Philadelphia, PA
Hahnemann Medical Center, Philadelphia, CA	University of Rochester, Rochester, NY
Harvard Medical School, Cambridge, MA	Yale Univ Hospital, New Haven, CT
Henry Ford Hospital, Detroit, MI	

The Daily Guide

Attending medical school classes are only a part of your life in Israel. Even in mysterious Israel, you will still need to use your hair dryer or listen to music or shop for food. The daily survival guide below lists some of the useful information you need to know about life in Israel.

Phone Calls Home
Dial 001+area code+phone number. Many students use ATT or other telephone company calling cards.

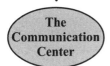

The Communication Center

Postal Service
Regular air-mails from Israel to U.S. require 2 shekels and postcards require 1.20 shekels. FEDEX service is available from Israel.

Fax Service
Students may fax from anywhere in Tel Aviv or the university campus.

Food & Supermarkets
There are plenty of regular supermarkets where students shop for food. Many shop at small fruit vendors or nut venders for snacks, and enjoy visiting the Shuk (Arab market) to get fresh fish, flowers, spices, you name it. It's a quick bus or a bike ride away.

Electricity Check
Israel's electrical supply is 220 volts and 50 hertz.

In Case Of Emergency

Contact
The American Embassy in Tel Aviv

or

The New York Office
(212) 688-8811

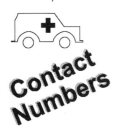

Contact Numbers

▶ **Live From Israel**

by Alanna Mishler

I am happy to say that I am truly enjoying my experience here. Since I worked as a nurse in the United States for five years, I feel that I have a good grasp of what the world of health care involves. I have many friends who have been through medical school or are currently going through the process in the United States. As a result, I have a basis for comparing Sackler's curriculum with any American medical school curriculum. The curriculum is basically the same as the standard U.S. ones. The differences you see are the same differences that exist between any American medical schools. Anatomy is a full year course here. The anatomy department has got to be one of the best in the world with professors who are not only anatomists, but anthropologists as well! The school is incredibly supportive. Because it is a foreign school, they make every effort to ensure excellent scores on the USMLE exams, including offering a semester long board review course during the second year. The school has excellent residency connections in both New York and California. There may be some difficulties obtaining residencies in other states, but determined students seem to manage it.

Classes are all taught in English, although some of the professors have heavy accents and are difficult to understand. My experiences in the American school system (Penn and UCLA) were the same, however. I appreciate finding out about the most recent research from all over the world and not just the United States. Early clinical exposure starts in the first year with students meeting a physician who sets up experiences in the hospital. Students often have the opportunity to participate in procedures that they would not be allowed to do in the United States, and therefore often find after graduation (according to graduates I have spoken to) that their clinical experience has been more comprehensive. Communication can be a barrier in the clinical setting, however. Thankfully, most Israelis speak English.

Tel Aviv is a modern, westernized city with all of the conveniences an American student would expect. Sackler is located at the Tel Aviv University. The school campus includes three swimming pools, basketball and tennis courts, racketball, and a gym with weight machines, stairmasters and treadmills. The city and University offer everything from movie theaters and museums to restaurants and clean beaches. Israel, of course, is full of historical sites as well.

That's all I can write for now – I must get to class. I love it here and feel at home. Some students find the stress of being far from home a bit much at times, but we are incredibly supportive of one another because we know we're all in the same situation. I hope you receive more information regarding this school because I think it deserves recognition!

In Their Own Words...

Comments From Current Sackler Medical Students

"Students often have the opportunity to participate in procedures that they would not be allowed to do in the United States, and therefore often find after graduation (according to graduates I have spoken to) that their clinical experience has been more comprehensive."

My Sackler Experience

by Scott Weiner (Sackler class of 1999)

Coming to school at Sackler was perhaps the best decision of my life, because it has been one of the most enriching and growing periods of my life so far. It has been wonderful to study medicine in an environment and culture that is new to me. Two years into the program and I know a hell of a lot about not only medicine, but also Israeli politics (which is perhaps a more impressive feat than learning medicine). In addition, I am slowly learning to speak Hebrew.

I think the most important suggestion that I can make to any pre-med student on whether or not to consider a foreign medical school is this: If you are not going into the experience with an open mind and a positive attitude, you should not attend a foreign medical school. Studying medicine is a huge commitment that requires monumental amounts of work. Being far away from one's family and friends, and having to cope and adjust to a new environment, make studying and succeeding all the more difficult. The only way to make the experience worthwhile is to have a positive attitude and an open mind to one's new surroundings.

Now for those students interested in attending Sackler. My main suggestion would be to try to study some Hebrew before coming to Israel. Although all lectures are in English, the first language of the patients and doctors you will work with is Hebrew. Understanding and being able to speak Hebrew at even a minimal level will give you worlds of insight during the clinical years in the hospitals. In addition, knowledge of Hebrew opens up the door to make Israeli friends and to break out of the "pseudocommunity" of English speaking medical school students. Again, Hebrew is not a requirement to attend school here. However, in my opinion, it would make life a whole lot easier.

As far as a list of what to consider when choosing a foreign medical school, I don't know what to say because Sackler was the only foreign medical school to which I applied.

Finally, due to the new "initiatives" to cut down on residencies in New York and Utah, I don't know if I would suggest a foreign medical school to anyone at this point. However, in another month we will see the residency match results for Sackler students. I am very interested to see how these new initiatives will affect foreign medical school graduates, and medical school graduates as a whole.

"I think the most important suggestion that I can make to any pre-med student on whether or not to consider a foreign medical school is this: If you are not going into the experience with an open mind and a positive attitude, you should not attend a foreign medical school."

The Caribbean Basin

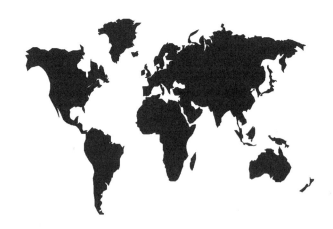

American University Of The Caribbean
School of Medicine

St. Maarten Campus
174 Defiance Road • Middle Region • St. Maarten
Netherlands Antilles

Medical Education Information Office
901 Ponce de Leon Blvd. #201 • Coral Gables • FL 33134
Phone: (305) 446-0600

The School Profile

The American University of the Caribbean (AUC) was founded in 1978 by Dr. Paul S. Tien. The University's School of Medicine was chartered by the Government of Montserrat and was approved by the Ministry of Education. AUC is listed in WHO's World Directory of Medical Schools.

AUC's campus is situated in Plymouth, Montserrat. The campus consists of approximately 17 buildings that house lecture halls, laboratories, and dormitories. According to AUC's brochure, "AUC's M.D. program has prepared close to 2,000 medical students to become caring, responsible, and compassionate medical doctors." The brochure also states that AUC graduates practices medicine in most U.S. states including California, Florida and New York.

AUC conducts all its basic sciences classes at the Monserrat campus. Clinical trainings are conducted at affiliated hospitals in the United States, England and other locations.

The AUC student-body hails from a wide variety of backgrounds. Along with traditional medical students, AUC also boasts a significant number of non-traditional students who may have already been practicing professionals in various allied health sciences professions.

According to AUC, most faculty members are American or British trained.

UPDATE: Due to recent volcanic activities on the island of Montserrat, AUC is now conducting its basic sciences curriculum at its St. Maarten campus in Netherlands Antilles.

Location

English is widely spoken in St. Maarten.

At the time of the printing of this book, AUC's basic sciences curriculum was being conducted in St. Maarten, Netherlands Antilles. St. Maarten is located approximately 150 miles east of Puerto Rico. The island is divided into two territories. The Dutch territory is referred to as St. Maarten while the French half is known as St. Martin. The AUC campus is located a few miles from the Dutch capital of Philipsburg.

Admission Requirements

3 entering classes per year:
January, May and September

The minimum admission requirements for applicants from North America (the United States and Canada) are as follows:

- A bachelor's degree from an accredited university or college prior to matriculation into the University is preferred. A minimum of 90 semester hours of college level work is required for admission.
- Completion of premedical curriculum that includes the following courses:
    1. General biology with laboratory – one year (two semesters)
    2. Inorganic chemistry with laboratory – one year (two semesters)
    3. Organic chemistry with laboratory – one year (two semesters)
    4. Physics with laboratory – one year (two semesters)
    5. English – one year (two semesters)

    Courses in mathematics, humanities and social sciences are recommended.
- OPTIONAL: Medical College Admission Test (MCAT) score. AUC strongly recommends applicants to sit for the MCAT.

Selection Factors

According to the official University brochure, "… the evaluation for admission is conducted on an individual basis. Students who enter the medical program are selected for their intellectual and social maturity…". In addition, the University considers problem-solving and critical judgment skills. Furthermore, the Admissions Committee also considers students' abilities to pursue independent study. Academic achievement, course load, difficulty of courses and major area of study are important factors in the selection process. Finally, non-academic factors such as motivation, maturity and personal integrity are also taken into consideration.

The Curriculum

The AUC M.D. program is 9½ semesters long. Required courses for graduation may be completed in 38 months if taken continuously. Each semester lasts for approximately 16 weeks.

The first five semesters of the M.D. program consist of courses in basic medical sciences. Students are required to enroll in various courses including Gross Anatomy, Biochemistry, Embryology, Cell Biology & Histology, Neuroscience, Genetics, and Physiology. All basic sciences courses are completed at AUC's Caribbean campus (currently located in St. Maarten).

The clinical sciences program is comprised of seventy-two weeks (4½ semesters) of clerkships at affiliated hospitals. The core clinical rotations are in Internal Medicine, Surgery, Pediatrics, Obstetrics & Gynecology and Psychiatry. Additionally, students are expected to complete 30 weeks of electives and courses in other clinical disciplines. All clinical rotations are completed at hospitals in the U.S., U.K. and other regions of the world.

Student Life

The climate of St. Maarten is pleasant throughout the year. As a result, biking, fishing, scuba diving and snorkeling are year-round activities available to students. Students participate in various on-campus student-run organizations including the Student Government Association and the Student Activities and Development Association. The official University brochure also states that "…students are eligible to join American Medical Student Association (AMSA)…".

Counseling, note and tutorial services are also available to students. A Spouses Club provides support to significant others of AUC medical students.

Residency Appointments

Internal Medicine

New Britain General Hospital
New Britain, CT
Danbury Hospital
Danbury, CT
Roger Williams Hospital
Providence, RI
Deaconess Hospital
St. Louis, MO
Univ of Nebraska Med. Cntr.
Omaha, NE

Veterans Affairs Medical Center
Salem, VA
Sinai Samaritan Medical Center
Milwaukee, WI
Hennepin Medical Center
Minneapolis, MN
St. Joseph Hospital & Medical Cntr.
Paterson, NJ
Staten Island University Hospital
Staten Island, NY

Family Practice

Deaconess Hospital
Evansville, IN

University of Louisville
Louisville, KY

Surgery

St. Joseph Mercy Hospital
Pontiac, MI

Mt. Sinai Medical Center
Elmhurst, NY

Pediatrics

St. John Hospital
Detroit, MI

Wayne State University
Detroit, MI

Students also obtained residencies in other specialties including Neurology, Psychiatry, Anesthesiology, Primary Care, Infectious Diseases, Vascular Surgery, Gastronomy, Pathology and Physical Medicine/Rehabilitation.

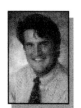

Dr. W. C. Stewart

B.S.–University of
Texas, Austin

M.D.–American
University of the
Caribbean School of
Medicine

*L*ife on the Rock
by William C. Stewart, M.D.

After finishing my undergraduate studies at the University of Texas in Austin, I came to the realization that my grade point average would not be sufficient enough to enable me to get into medical school. I applied to several medical schools in Texas, and around the country, with the same end result. Getting into an American medical school was, at the time, extremely competitive, much like it is today. Without having an A average and an immaculate resume, the chance was slim. I was considering changing majors from Chemistry to Advertising.

I received a letter from my grandfather, who sent with it a newspaper clip from USA Today, about a Caribbean medical school called The American University of the Caribbean. I was skeptical, but called the number to receive the brochure. After months of deliberating I decided to call the island of Montserrat, where the school was located. I spoke with several faculty members and a few students. A few weeks later I was on a plane headed towards the British West Indies for an impromptu meeting. My main concerns were whether AUC was accredited by the World Health Organization, and if it was truly a school and not some hoax. It was during this time that Caribbean medical schools were getting bad publicity for basically handing out diplomas to students who hadn't attended one. This was, obviously, a situation that I did not want to find myself getting into.

The basic outline of the academic schedule for AUC was pretty simple. I must spend the first year and a half on the island completing my basic science courses, and then on to Detroit, or England, for the clerkships. The entrance requirements for AUC were pretty simple, if you have the money, they'll take you. There was very little interest in academic grades or MCAT scores.

After looking around the campus and meeting the faculty, I realized that this was a real school and not just some phony scam. I spoke with the students and everyone seemed to be very homesick, but also very serious about becoming an MD. The professors were slightly over qualified. Two were retired from Harvard, and lived on the island and played golf everyday after their classes. Several others were retired teachers and M.D.'s from other schools in the U.S. The student population was diverse. Though low in numbers, there was a smorgasbord of personalities. There were older students, retired pharmacists, optometrists and students of all race and color.

I applied, handed AUC a check for the first semester, and off I went. The dorm rooms were average, and were cooled by ceiling fans. We were without electricity, and fresh water for more than a week. The natives in

Montserrat grew restless and began looting the downtown stores and shops. I was hoping that this disaster would help me get into an American medical school. The rumors of St. George students being transferred to American schools after the Grenada incident began to fly. But no such luck. After 8 days of living like animals, with contact through HAM radio to the outside world, we were finally picked up by the U.S. Coast Guard and brought to Antigua where we then managed to fly home. I waited for almost two months, unsure what the school had planned for us. I heard rumors that the owner of the school had recently dropped the insurance on the school and was just going to cut his losses and close it down. I went to the Texas medical schools and asked if they would consider me for transfer, and they all said no. Finally I heard the news. We were all going to Plainview, Texas to finish the rest of our basic science courses while the school was rebuilt on the island. The entire staff and crew were sent to Plainview, and I finished my basic science days in the panhandle. The day I was done, the AUC was rebuilt and the rest of the students had to move back to the island.

I started my clinical rotations at Kingston Hospital in England. During my stay in England, I was also cramming for the National Board Exam. I passed the exam and then finished my elective courses at the University of Texas. I graduated from AUC in three and a half years and went back to the island for graduation. I took my family with me, so that they could see first hand what I had to overcome. The number of students in my graduating class had dwindled from 40 to about 13, and some of these students I had never seen before, as they were from previous class years.

I had my diploma from AUC, but was not exactly the proudest of people. I was an M.D., but was embarrassed to tell people were I had gone to medical school. I managed to pull some strings and talk to the internal medicine program at the University of Texas Medical Branch in Galveston. They said they would take me into the Internal Medicine program if I passed my National Boards Part II. I did, and they took me in. I later managed to be in the right place at the right time to find an Ophthalmology program that would accept me. I took the position and finished up with a fellowship in Oculoplastic surgery.

Now, life is good. I was surfing the internet the other night for Caribbean Medical Schools. I found a few links to webpages and some general information, but did not, however, find any information on AUC. Since I graduated from medical school, the island was hit with another disaster. The volcano began to erupt and made headline news around the world. The students were moved to another island where I believe the beaches are white and not black. AUC has been through a lot and continues to rebound. I have heard that the census is up, owing to the ever increasing numbers of medical school applicants to U.S. medical schools.

The stigma of going to a Caribbean medical school will always be with me, but the further you get in your training the less and less people will ask you where you went to medical school. I wanted to submit this article for people who are considering going to medical school outside of the U.S. It is not easy. There is a lot of prejudice toward foreign medical graduates, but there is a light at the end of the tunnel for those who can stick with it. The majority of my classmates dropped out and went back to their old jobs. Some students had nervous breakdowns, but a few, like myself, stuck it out and finished medical school. I am now a Board Certified Ophthalmologist practicing in Tennessee, and my roommate at AUC is a practicing Pathologist. Stick with it, and your dream can come true.

Saba University
School of Medicine

Saba Campus
P.O. Box 1000 • Saba • Netherlands Antilles
Phone: 011-599-463456 • Fax: 011-599-463458

Education Information Consultants, Inc.
P.O. Box 386 • Gardner • FL MA 01440
Phone: (508) 630-5122 • Fax: (508) 632-2168
E-mail: SABA@TIAC.NET

The School Profile

Saba University School of Medicine was organized in 1986 as a collaborative effort between the island government of Saba and a group of medical educators from the United States. In 1988, Saba University was approved by the Government of the Netherland Antilles and an official operating charter was granted by the Government of Saba in October 1992. In mid-1994, Saba University's Board of Trustees adopted a Bachelor of Science degree program in Medical Science and a Master of Science degree in Hyperbaric Medicine.

Saba University School of Medicine is listed in the World Directory of Medical Schools by the WHO.

Location

The offical language of Saba is Dutch. English is spoken widely.

The island of Saba was discovered by Columbus on his second voyage to the New World, in the late 1400s. Since then Saba has been ruled by the English, French, and Spanish. However, during the last two hundred years the Saba has remained a Dutch island. Saba is a five square mile island in the northeastern Caribbean, 28 miles south of St. Maarten. Together with Statia, these three islands form the Windward Islands of the Dutch Caribbean. Saba is known as "The Unspoiled Queen" because of all the rich, tropical, natural beauty present on the island. At 2,800 feet above the sea level, a dense rain forest often peeks out from behind a light, cool cloud.

The daytime temperature on Saba averages 80°F. Year-round Easterly trade winds create ever changing cloud movements. The average minimum annual rainfall on the island is 42 inches.

Admission Requirements

There is no set deadline for admissions.

The minimum admission requirements for applicants from North America (the United States and Canada) are listed below. However, the University adds that "...students may deviate from these criteria and still qualify for admission to the M.D. program...".

■ A bachelor's degree from an accredited university or college prior to matriculation into the University is recommended. A minimum of 90 semester hours or 135 quarter hours of college/university work must be completed.
■ Completion of premedical curriculum that includes the following courses:
    1. General biology with laboratory – three years (six semesters)
    2. Inorganic chemistry with laboratory – one year (two semesters)
    3. Organic chemistry with laboratory – one year (two semesters)
    4. Physics with laboratory – one semester (optional)

■ Applicants whose native language is not English are required to take the TOEFL.

Selection Factors

According to the official University brochure, "...the Committee on Admissions will select those applicants whom they judge to be the best qualified for the study and practice of medicine. The committee will consider evidence of intellectual curiosity, emotional maturity, honesty, and proper motivation in addition to proven scholastic ability...".

Saba University's School of Medicine receives approximately 2000 applicants for the 30 to 35 positions available in each entering classes.

The Curriculum

The total time required to complete the M.D. program is 40 months (with out summer breaks). With summer breaks included, the program is 48 months long. The basic science program is five semesters long. It takes approximately 20 months to complete. The basic sciences curriculum includes courses in Gross Anatomy, Histology, Medical Embryology, Physiology, Biochemistry, Pharmacology and Medical Genetics. The basic sciences courses are completed at Saba's basic science campus which is located immediately adjacent to the A. M. Edwards Medical Center.

The clinical medicine program lasts for 72 weeks. Clinical rotations are completed in affiliated hospitals in the United States, Saba, St. Martin and Curacao. Students spend 42 weeks completing required core rotations in Internal Medicine, Surgery, Obstetrics and Gynecology, Pediatrics, and Psychiatry. Additional 30 weeks are devoted to elective clinical rotations.

University of Health Sciences Antigua
School of Medicine

Downhill Campus
P.O. Box 510 • St. John's • Antigua
West Indies
Phone: (809) 460-1391 • Fax: (809) 460-1477

The School Profile

The University of Health Sciences Antigua (UHSA) School of Medicine was established in 1982. UHSA is a privately owned medical school. It is chartered by the Government of Antigua and Barbuda. The campus is approximately 50 acres in size and lies entirely within the Historical National Park area of English Harbor. UHSA is also listed in the World Directory of Medical Schools by the WHO.

According to the University brochure, "…recent graduates from the University of Health Sciences Antigua School of Medicine have served in residencies in major health care and teaching facilities in all parts of the United States…". In addition the school adds that "…the medical school endeavors to recruit faculty members with significant interests and achievements in research…".

It is important to note that UHSA does not administer any loan or scholarship assistance programs. UHSA students are not eligible for U.S. government sponsored loan programs such as the Stafford Loan. All students must pay in full upon acceptance into UHSA's M.D. program.

Location

English is the official language of Antigua.

The island of Antigua is located in the Eastern Caribbean. It is approximately 3 hours away from Miami. Antigua is approximately 110 square miles in area and tropical in nature. It was discovered by Columbus in 1493 and since then the Spanish, French and English have fought over this tiny island. Except for a short period of time, Antigua has remained under British authority. Currently, Antigua is a monarchy of the British Queen.

The temperature ranges between 76°F and 85°F throughout the year. The average annual rainfall on the island is 45 inches. Antigua is famous for its world-renowned coral reefs and beaches. In fact, more than 300 beaches exist in Antigua.

Admission Requirements

The minimum admission requirements for applicants from North America (the United States and Canada) are listed below. However, the University adds that "...the academic committee has no preference for a major field of undergraduate study."

- A bachelor's degree from an accredited university or college prior to matriculation into the University is recommended.
- Completion of premedical curriculum that includes the following courses:
    1. General biology with laboratory – one year (two semesters)
    2. Inorganic chemistry with laboratory – one year (two semesters)
    3. Organic chemistry with laboratory – one year (two semesters)
    4. English – one year (two semesters)

- OPTIONAL: Medical College Admissions Test (MCAT) score.

Selection Factors

Information not available.

The Curriculum

The total time required to complete the M.D. program at UHSA is four years.. Like U.S. medical schools, the medical curriculum at UHSA is segmented into two years of basic sciences studies followed by two years of clinical work.

During the first year, UHSA medical students complete courses in Anatomy, Biochemistry, Embryology, Genetics, Histology, Medical Terminology, Nutrition, Physiology and Introduction to Clinical Practice Part I.

The second basic sciences year consists of courses in Biostatistics, Immunology, Pathology, Neurosciences, Medical Microbiology, Medical Jurisprudence, Pharmacology, Physical Diagnosis, and Introduction to Clinical Practice Part II.

The third and fourth year of the M.D. program is devoted to clinical training. Clinical training involves rotations in various medical disciplines. At the time of the printing of this book, no information was available regarding the location of clinical training or affiliated hospitals.

Universidad Iberoamericana
School of Medicine

Av. Francia 129 • Santo Domingo • Dominican Republic
Phone: (809) 689-4111 • Fax: (809) 686-5821 or (809) 686-5533

UNIBE, ID# 10459
P.O. Box 025577 • Miami • FL 33102-5577
Phone: 1-800-203-3562 (USA) or 1-900-265-3266 (Canada)
E-mail: unibe.adm@codetel.net.do

The School Profile

The Iberoamerican University or Universidad Iberoamericana (UNIBE) was established in 1982 in Santo Domingo, Dominican Republic. UNIBE is a private, non-sectarian university. The University includes Schools of Law, Business, Architecture, Marketing, Theorlogy, Arts, and Dentistry and Medicine.

The UNIBE School of Medicine is located in the center of Santo Domingo. The campus is surrounded by the city's major governmental buildings, museums, art galleries and theaters. The campus is also surrounded by tropical gardens.

The medical curriculum at the School of Medicine is conducted in English. However, students are expected to enroll in Spanish classes in order to better interact with Spanish speaking patients and personnel of the University.

Location

The population of Dominican Republic is 8 million.

The country of Dominican Republic is located between the islands of Cuba and Puerto Rico in the Caribbean Sea. Dominican Republic shares the island known as Hispaniola with Haiti. The country is approximately 18,700 square miles in size. Its primary language is Spanish.

Santo Domingo, the capital of Dominican Republic, is one of the oldest cities in the western hemisphere. The climate of the city is warm and tropical. The average temperature is 77°F. Like most Caribbean islands, Dominican Republic is swept by warm trade winds year round.

Admission Requirements

The minimum admission requirements for applicants from North America (the United States and Canada) are listed below.

- A bachelor's degree from an accredited university or college prior to matriculation into the University is recommended. However, the University requires completion of at least 90 semester hours of college work.
- Completion of premedical curriculum that includes the following courses:
    1. General biology with laboratory – one year (two semesters)
    2. Inorganic chemistry with laboratory – one year (two semesters)
    3. Organic chemistry with laboratory – one semester
    4. Mathematics with Calculus – one year (two semesters)
    5. Physics with laboratory – one year (two semesters)

- OPTIONAL: Medical College Admissions Test (MCAT) score.

Selection Factors

According to the University, "…admissions to our School of Medicine requires that candidates possess certain personal traits: maturity, responsibility, emotional stability, academic ability and integrity." Usually, an interview is conducted with most applicants to the School of Medicine.

The Curriculum

Students must attend 80% of classes in any given course in order to sit for the final examination.

Iberoamericana University's medical program is composed of 11 semesters lasting 176 weeks. Each semester is 16 weeks long. The first five of the 11 semesters are dedicated to basic sciences courses. The basic sciences curriculum consists of several courses including classes in Gross Anatomy, Biochemistry, Histology, Physiology, Parasitology, Behavior Sciences, Pathology, Microbiology, and Forensic Medicine.

Clinical work is completed during the remaining duration of the medical program. As part of the clinical curriculum, students complete rotations in Internal Medicine, Pediatrics, Surgery, Obstetrics and Gynecology and Psychiatry. Students are also required to complete numerous elective seminars including Tropical Medicine, Child Abuse and Health Management.

All clinical rotations are completed in UNIBE's own hospitals as well as in six affiliated hospitals. The following is a list of hospitals where students perform their clinical clerkships:
- National Institute for Diabetes, Endocrinology & Nutrition
- Dr. Robert Read Children's Hospital
- National Institute of Cardiology
- M.E. Perdomo Maternity Hospital
- H. Pieter Oncological Institute

Spartan Health Sciences University
School of Medicine

P.O. Box 324 • Vieux Fort • St. Lucia • West Indies
Phone: (758) 454-6128 • Fax: (758) 454-6811

U.S. Information Office
6500 Boeing Drive, Suite L-201 • El Paso • TX 79925
Phone: (915) 778-5309 or (915) 778-5310 or (915) 778-5327
Fax: (915) 778-5328

The School Profile

Spartan Health Sciences University School of Medicine was established in St. Lucia on January 7, 1980. The University was chartered by the Government of St. Lucia and is listed in the World Directory of Medical Schools.

Location

St. Lucia's Head of State is Queen Elizabeth II of England.

The island of St. Lucia is located in the eastern Caribbean. It is the second largest island in the Windward Island chain. The country is approximately 283 square miles in size. St. Lucia is tropical in nature. The weather is warm and mildly humid year round.

The official language of the island is English. However, a large number of residents also converse in French patois. The population of the country is approximately 150,000. Most people reside in the port cities of Castries and Vieux Fort.

Admission Requirements

3 entering classes per year:
January, May and September

The minimum admission requirements for applicants from North America (the United States and Canada) are listed below.

- A bachelor's degree from an accredited university or college prior to matriculation into the University is recommended. A minimum requirement for admission to the School of Medicine is 90 semester hours of college level work.

- Completion of premedical curriculum that includes the following courses:
    1. General biology with laboratory – one year (two semesters)
    2. Inorganic chemistry with laboratory – one year (two semesters)
    3. Organic chemistry with laboratory – one year (two semesters)
    4. Physics with laboratory – one year (two semesters)

- Required courses must have been taken no more than five years prior to application for admission. A cumulative average of B or better is recommened in required courses.

Selection Factors

Information not available.

The Curriculum

The M.D. program at Spartan University is 36 months long (three years). Classes are held on a trimester basis. Each trimester lasts for four months. The program is divided into two segments — basic medical sciences and clinical sciences. The first 16 months are devoted to basic medical sciences while the next 20 months cover the clinical sciences. Clinical training is hospital based, however, the locations of affiliated hospitals are not known.

Mexico

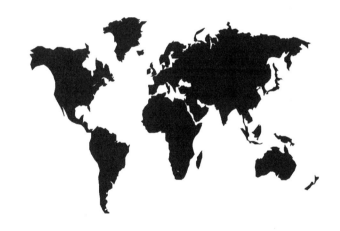

Universidad Autonoma de Guadalajara
School of Medicine

Av. Patria 1201
Guadalajara • Jaslico • Mexico

UAG Office in the United States
8801 Callaghan Road • San Antonio • TX 78230-4417
Phone: (800) 531-5494 or (210) 366-1611
Fax: (210) 377-2975
E-mail: iep@txdirect.net • *Internet: http://www.gdl.uag.mx*

The School Profile

Universidad Autonoma de Guadalajara (UAG) was founded in 1935. It is the oldest and largest private university in Mexico. UAG offers approximately 49 undergraduate, 26 master and 2 doctorate degrees. The University is accredited by the Mexican Federal Department of Public Education.

UAG boasts over twenty schools including schools of Agriculture, Biological Sciences, Fine Arts, Law, Nursing and Engineering. UAG's School of Medicine is primarily composed of Mexican students, although a significant number of foreign students come from the United States, Canada and Puerto Rico. According to the University brochure nearly 8,000 physicians who obtained their medical training at the UAG are practicing in the U.S., Canada and Puerto Rico.

UAG's on-campus holdings include two teaching hospitals, three convention centers, four libraries, a publishing facility, and a television studio. In addition, support facilities such as a bank, automatic tellers, a copy center, a post office, a sports shop, a gasoline station, and a book shop are also found on-campus. In addition, UAG boasts the International Languages Center and the Center for Asian and Latin American Studies.

Location

The temperature in Guadalajara ranges between 75°F and 100°F

Guadalajara is the capital of the Mexican state Jalisco. The city was founded by Nuno De Guzman in 1542. Guadalajara stands at a height of 5,000 feet above sea level on the Pacific Coast of Western Mexico. The near perfect warm weather of Guadalajara has attracted more than 5 million people as permanent residents. A large American population resides in or near the city as well.

The city is characterized by its numerous tree-lined boulevards and avenues. It is not uncommon to see flowers such as carnations and jasmine flourish next to lemon and orange trees in various corners of

Guadalajara. Guadalajara is one of Mexico's most historically and culturally rich cities. Numerous museums and theaters are found throughout the city.

Admission Requirements

2 entering classes per year:
January and August

The minimum admission requirements for applicants from North America (the United States and Canada) are the following:

- A bachelor's degree from an accredited university or college prior to matriculation into the University is preferred. A minimum of 90 semester hours of college level work is required for admission.
- Completion of premedical curriculum that includes the following courses:
    1. General biology with laboratory – eight semester credit hours
    2. Inorganic chemistry with laboratory – eight semester credit hours
    3. Organic chemistry with laboratory – eight semester credit hours
    4. Physics with laboratory – eight semester credit hours

- OPTIONAL: Medical College Admission Test (MCAT) score.

Selection Factors

According to the official University brochure, "…the Committee on University Admissions (of Foreign Students) to the School of Medicine requires applicants to have a 3.00 cumulative grade-point average and above average scores on the MCAT." However, the admissions committee adds that "…the simple review of numbers is not a sufficient indicator of an applicant's potential to become a good physician." Students whose academic records are less than stellar must demonstrate other qualities in order to receive a favorable decision from the Admissions Committee. The Committee weighs personal qualities such as maturity, ethical standards, and industriousness in their decision making process.

The Curriculum

The UAG medical curriculum is six years in length. The first four years are dedicated to traditional basic sciences courses followed by clinical training. The fifth year is composed of an internship which is followed by a year of social service. However, American citizens may complete the curriculum in four years and then enter the Fifth Pathway program in the United States before applying for ACGME-approved residency programs.

All students who enter the Fifth Pathway program *must* post a monetary bond with the university. The University brochure states the following:
"The student must also post a bond, which is forfeited if he or she does not

return to Mexico for the year of Social Service. These funds, if forfeited, are then used to help support community medicine programs for the underprivileged."

The medical school also maintains two special programs – the International Program and the Co-op Program for American students.

All foreign students including U.S. citizens are also required to pass tests related to Mexican government, geography and history. Short two week didactic courses covering the above mentioned subjects are conducted by the University for the benefit of medical students. Passing grades must be obtained in all three areas within one year of enrollment.

Teaching Facilities

The UAG School of Medicine maintains two separate campuses – the Institute of Biological Sciences (ICB) and Dr. Angel Leano University Hospital and Medical Center (HAL). The first two years of the medical curriculum are carried out at the ICB facility. The next two clinical years are completed at the HAL Medical Center.

ICB campus is located approximately a mile from the central university campus. ICB contains laboratories, libraries and other supporting facilities. The University Hospital and Medical Center is five miles away from the central campus nestled in the hills surrounding the city of Guadalajara. Located within the Medical Center are a large teaching hospital, clinical laboratories, lecture halls and numerous classrooms.

Financial Aid

U.S. citizens enrolled full-time at UAG School of Medicine qualify for various financial aid packages. In the past, UAG students were eligible for various federal loan programs including the Stafford and Supplemental Loans. Please check with the UAG Financial Aid Office (1-800-531-5494) for the most up-to-date information on financial aid packages. It is important to note that Mexico was **not** one of the four countries identified by the U.S. Department of Education whose medical programs were "comparable to those used to evaluate programs leading to the M.D. degree in the United States." Please be aware that the U.S. Department of Education's accreditation standards may affect a school's eligibility for various federal loan programs.

Eastern Europe

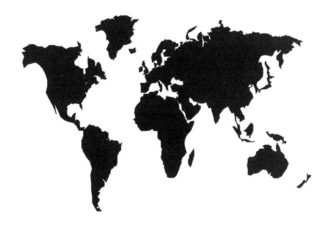

Karol Marcinkowski University
of Medical Sciences

Poznan • Poland
US Office: Corvestor Services Corporation
11 Market Street, Suite 204 • Poughkeepsie • NY 12601
Phone: (914) 454-5151 • Fax: (914) 454-6612
Internet: http://som.flinders.edu.au/ • E-mail: dwl2@usoms.poznan.pl

---

The School Profile

Karol Marcinkowski University of Medical Sciences (MUMS) has been serving the Polish medical community for many years. The University is comprised of ten institutes, forty-four departments, and seventeen chairs in the Medical Faulty. In addition, the University cooperates with sixteen other research institutions worldwide. MUMS is accredited by the Ministry of Health and Social Welfare of the Republic of Poland.

In 1950, the Medical Faculty with the section of Dentistry and the Faculty of Pharmacy were detached to form an independent school – the University of Medical Sciences in Poznan, In 1975, the nursing school was established. Four years later, the Section of Medical Analytics was formed. In 1984, the Polish Parliament conferred upon the University its present name – Karol Marcinkowski University of Medical Sciences. In 1992, Medical Faculty II was established. The current four-year English language Medical Program is run under the auspices of Medical Faculty II. The first class in the four year English language Medical Program is scheduled to graduate in 1997.

According to the University, between the years 1950 and 1994 the Medical School has granted more than 11,000 *Dyplom Lekarz* (academic medical diploma) degrees. The school also adds that there are more than 1600 medical students of which 139 were non-Poles.

Location

The city of Poznan is located on the banks of River Warta in Western Poland. Poznan is an historic town that has existed for over 1,000 years. Approximately 700,000 people inhabit the city. Poznan is the gateway city between Berlin and Warsaw.

Poznan is a city full of greenery and lakes. The pleasant environment of the city is enhanced by the presence of a picturesque medieval downtown area. Poznan also serves as a center for European trade and industrial conventions throughout the year.

Admission Requirements

The minimum admission requirements for applicants from North America (the United States and Canada) are the following:

- A bachelor's degree from an accredited university or college prior to matriculation into the University.
- Completion of premedical curriculum that includes the following courses:
    1. General biology with laboratory – one year (two semesters)
    2. Inorganic chemistry with laboratory – one year (two semesters)
    3. Organic chemistry with laboratory – one year (two semesters)
    4. Physics with laboratory – one year (two semesters)
    5. English – one year (two semesters)
- OPTIONAL: Medical College Admission Test (MCAT) score

Selection Factors

According to the University brochure, "…the University seeks individuals with broad educational backgrounds…" However, the University also states that each applicant must demonstrate a record of academic achievement. The Admissions Committee seeks individuals who have the ability to master scientific concepts as well as those with personal traits compatible with practice of medicine. The University seeks to admit mature individuals who are prepared to handle the rigors of medical school.

The Curriculum

The four year medical program at MUMS in Poznan is designed for American and Canadian college graduates who have completed their premedical education. The program is taught in English although Polish is gradually introduced to enable students work in clinics.

Like most four year curriculum, the first two years are dedicated to basic sciences while the last two years are for clinical training. A total of 2,010 hours of didactic instruction is imparted to students during basic sciences years. Clinical training takes place at the five State Clinical Hospitals and other affiliated hospitals in Poznan.

Financial Aid

MUMS does not offer scholarships to students intending to study medicine at Poznan. U.S. citizens may apply for Federal loans such as the Stafford Loan to finance their medical education.

Palacký University
Faculty of Medicine

Olomouc • Czech Republic
US Office: Palacky University Medical School USA, Inc.
1334 Walnut Street • Philadelphia • PA 19107
Phone: (215) 732-7943 • Fax: (610) 284-6960
E-mail: PALACKYMED@aol.com • dekanlf@risc.upol.cz

The School Profile

Palacký University was founded by Emperor Maximillian and Pope Gregor XIII in 1573. The University is located in the city of Olomouc, in the Czech Republic. Among many things, the University is known as the home of the famous founder of modern genetics, Johann Gregor Mendel.

After years of success and decline, the University was reopened in 1946 and was named after František Palacký. At the present, Palacký is home to more than 11,000 students enrolled in all seven colleges of the University.

The Medical Faculty of Palacký University is one of the seven colleges of the University. The medical school is listed in the WHO's Directory of Medical Schools. Students at Palacký may study medicine in either Czech or English. According to the University, "…in the forty year period from 1957 to 1996, 450 students from many countries such as Germany, Greece, Israel, Jordan, Korea, Kuwait, Poland, Sudan and Yemen have earned medical degrees here." The University also states that more than eighty students are studying in the English Language program at Palacký University. Students in the English Language program hail from countries like Great Britain, India, Jordan, and the United States.

Location

Olomouc, a town of medium size, is located in the fertile basin of the Morava River in the central Moravia region of the Czech Republic. Not far from the town of Olomouc lies the Jeseníky Mountains, a favorite place of skiers, hikers and campers. Olomouc boasts a population of approximately 120,000 people. The town is a center for various cultural, business, and religious activities. The city's architecture is one of the best in the country. Olomouc is also the proud home of the Moravian Philharmonic Orchestra and the Moravian Theater. The climate of Olomouc is mild and the temperature averages between 25° Celsius in the summer and 0° Celsius in the winter.

Admission Requirements

The minimum admission requirements for applicants from North America (the United States and Canada) are the following:

- A bachelor's degree from an accredited university or college prior to matriculation into the University.

- OPTIONAL: Medical College Admission Test (MCAT) score

Selection Factors

Information Not Available.

The Curriculum

The medical program at Palacký University is *six* years long. All lectures and tests are conducted in English. However, the framework of the curriculum is similar to the program designed for Czech medical students. As a result, learning the Czech language is a mandatory requirement for all students in the English Language program.

The curriculum is divided into three parts called "rigorosa." The first part covers the concepts and fundamentals of basic sciences over a four semester period. The second part is dedicated to the learning of the disease state with introduction to basic clinical sciences. The last part deals with clinical medicine and the practice of medicine in hospital settings. Upon successful completion of all three parts of the program, students are awarded Medical Doctor's degree (MUDr.).

All instructions are conducted at either the Theoretical Institutes Building or the Faculty Hospital. The hospital is a large teaching institution with more than 1,800 beds for patients. It is a combination of many old and new facilities. For the most part, difficult disciplines such as surgical clinics, occupy the newer facilities.

Financial Aid

Palacký University does not offer scholarships to students intending to study medicine at their school. U.S. citizens attending Palacký are not eligible for Federal loans such as the Stafford Loan.

University Medical School of Debrecen
Debreceni Orvos Tudomanyi Egyetem (DOTE)

Debrecen• Hungary
H-4003 Debrecen • PO Box 4 • Hungary
Phone: 011-36-20-430-492 • Fax: 011-36-52-439-579
US Office: Tina's Medical Student Agency
130 3 E. 9th Street #2 • Upland • CA 91786
Phone: (909) 949-8399 • Fax: (909) 949-8399

The School Profile

The University at Debrecen was officially established in 1918. At its inception, the University was comprised of four colleges – Arts, Sciences, Theology, and Medicine. The current facilities of the medical schools including hospitals were constructed between 1926 and 1930. For many years, the medical school operated as an integral part of the University. However, in 1951 the medical school became independent from the University and started to operate as its own entity.

Currently, the medical school operated under the supervision of Hungary's Ministry of Health. The school has 21 basic sciences and 18 clinical sciences departments. In addition, the medical school has numerous affiliated hospitals throughout Hungary.

Location

Debrecen is the economic and cultural hub of Eastern Hungary. It is a city filled with tradition and history. After Budapest, Debrecen is the second largest city in Hungary. The city is an attraction for tourists as well as nature lovers. The natural thermal baths and spas are one of Debrecen's many assets. In addition, the city is surrounded by acres of forest land. Just outside the city limits is one of Hungary's great national parks, The Hortobágy National Park.

Debrecen is also a university town, with numerous universities and colleges located in the city. Some of them include the University Medical School, The Lajos Kossuth University of Arts and Sciences, the Teacher Training School, and the Reformed Academy of Theology.

Acording to the current American students at Debrecen, there are two McDonald's located in the city. A wholesale store similar to Sam's or Price Club is also found there. The word on Debrecen from current students: "…Debrecen is not a completely a boring place to live…"

Admission Requirements

The minimum admission requirements for applicants from North America (the United States and Canada) are the following:

- Passing scores on University administered entrance examinations.

- Previous knowledge of biology, chemistry, and physics is desirable.

- Medical College Admission Test (MCAT) score is not required.

Selection Factors

The University administers entrance examinations in biology, chemistry, and physics. The maximum score on the examination is 400 points. Each year the Vice Rector for Educational Affairs of the University determines the minimum scores needed to be admitted to the first-year class. Applicants may be exempted from entrance examinations if they have completed some courses in biology, chemistry and physics at accredited universities. No further information is available regarding selection factors from the University.

The Curriculum

The English Language program at Debrecen is *six* years long. The general medicine program is comprised of twelve semesters. Like most programs, the first two years are designed to teach students the concepts and fundamentals of basic sciences. During the third year, the students study basics of diseases. The next two years involve clinical rotations at the University affiliated hospitals. During the sixth and final year, students complete more rotations in internal medicine, surgery, gynecology, neurology, and pediatrics. Students are also expected to complete a senior thesis during their sixth year at the medical school.

Financial Aid

The University at Debrecen does not offer scholarships to students intending to study medicine at their school. According to the University, U.S. citizens attending Debrecen are eligible for Federal loans such as the Stafford Loan. However, in a recent US Department of Education survey, Hungary was not one of the countries approved for Federal Student Loans. Please check with the Department of Education in Washington, DC for the latest information.

Albert Szent-Györgyi Medical University
Szeged

Szeged• Hungary
Dean's Office • Albert Szent-Györgyi Med. University
H-6701 • PO Box 481 • Zrínyi U. 9 • Hungary
Internet: http://www.szote.u-szeged.hu

The School Profile

The Albert Szent-Györgyi Medical University was established in Kolozsvár, Transylvania in 1872. At the end of World War I, the University was relocated to the city of Szeged. Since then the medical school has served as the primary health care center for southern Hungary. The University is named after a former professor of the medical school, Prof. Albert Szent-Györgyi, who was the recepient of Noble Prize in Medicine in 1937.

The medical school or the Faculty of Medicine is located near the Cathedral Square in Szeged. The Faculty of Medicine building houses the preclinical departments of the medical school. The affiliated university hospitals are located between the Cathedral and the Tisza River. Some of the clinical departments are located in the University hospitals.

Location

Szeged is located in the south of Hungary. The city is a quaint town steeped in tradition and culture. River Tisza has long been the life of the city. The temperate summer and cold winters are common in this area of Hungary.

Admission Requirements

The minimum admission requirements for applicants from North America (the United States and Canada) are the following:

■ Must be a high school graduate.

■ Previous knowledge of biology, chemistry and physics.

■ Medical College Admission Test (MCAT) score is not required.

Selection Factors

An entrance examination is administered for all foreign applicants. In addition, all foreign applicants must show adequate mastery of the English language. No further information is available regarding selection factors.

The Curriculum

The medical program at Albert Szent-Györgyi Medical University is *six* years long. During the first two years, the curriculum concentrates on teaching basic sciences. The next three years are devoted to teaching both preclinical and clinical sciences. Students conclude the curriculum by completing clinical clerkships at University affiliated hospitals during the sixth year. At the end of the program, students must pass a series of final examinations in internal medicine, pediatrics, surgery, OB/GYN, psychiatry, and neurology. All clinical training takes place in the wards of clinical departments, outpatient clinics, and affiliated teaching hospitals.

Financial Aid

Albert Szent-Györgyi Medical University does not offer scholarships to students intending to study medicine at their school. U.S. citizens attending Szent-Györgyi Medical University are not eligible for Federal loans such as the Stafford Loan.

The United Kingdom

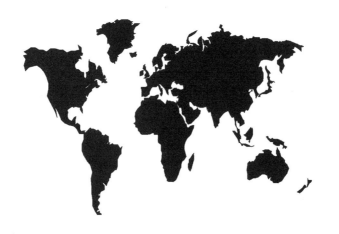

Kigezi International School of Medicine
Cambridge Overseas Medical Training Program

Director of Admissions
Kigezi International School of Medicine, Kabale
Cambridge Overseas Medical Training Program
181a Huntingdon Road • Cambridge CB3 0DJ • United Kingdom
Phone: 011-44-1223-327282 • Fax: 011-44-1223-324232
Internet: http://dialspace.dial.pipex.com/kigezi.med/
E-mail: kigezi.med@dial.pipex.com

The School Profile

Kigezi International School of Medicine is located in Uganda, Africa. Kigezi International School of Medicine is a tax-exempt non-governmental charity organization registered in the Republic of Uganda.

According to the school brochure, "…Kigezi International School of Medicine aims to train physicians with sound backgrounds in the basic medical sciences and a commitment to primary health care. A primary objective of Kigezi International School of Medicine is to provide invaluable training for international students in tropical medicine." The school further states that one of its other goals is to augment the medical resources of Uganda, particularly the region of Kigezi.

The pre-clinical instruction is conducted by the Cambridge Overseas Medical Training Program, located in the Cambridge Research Laboratories at the University of Cambridge, England. On the other hand, Clinical training is conducted in Uganda and on a limited basis in the United States. It is important to note that Kigezi International School of Medicine is in no way affiliated with the University of Cambridge.

Location

Cambridge has been an important settlement and market for more than 900 years. The City's continued growth was fostered with the establishment of the University in the 13th century; Peterhouse, the oldest college, was founded in 1284. The medieval colleges were all built in or beside the existing town whilst the more modern colleges are found mainly in the west of the City.

With its 108,000 residents (including 10,000 students) it is not a large city, but it is no longer just an East Anglian County town and historic university city. The western part of East Anglia is one of the fastest growing areas of Britain and looks to Cambridge as its sub-regional center for business, employment, shopping and leisure services.

Admission Requirements

Classes start three times a year: January, September & April

The minimum admission requirements for applicants from North America (the United States and Canada) are as follows:

- A bachelor's degree from an accredited university or college.

- A minimum of one year of study of biology and biochemistry.

- Medical College Admission Test (MCAT) score is required.

Selection Factors

Information Not Available.

The Curriculum

The medical program at Kigezi International is completed over four years. The program is designed in a manner that will enable U.S. citizens to successfully pass the USMLE and to qualify to practice medicine in the United States. *(Note: At the time of this printing, the publisher was not able to obtain the latest USMLE pass rate of Kigezi students).*

During the first two years of the program, students complete pre-clinical basic science courses at the Cambridge Research Laboratories of the University of Cambridge (England). Under the guidance from the Cambridge Overseas Medical Training Program, students complete all courses in England. While in Cambridge, students are housed at Westminister College – a traditional Cambridge College, located at the center of the town. All courses are taught by faculty composed primarily of University of Cambridge Lecturers, Tutors and Scholars.

The seventy-five weeks of clinical training are divided amongst clinical sites in Uganda (Africa) and the U.S. Students must spend six months training at Kabale Hospital in Uganda. Kabale Hospital is a 220-bed teaching hospital and is the sole provider of medical care for the entire region of Kigezi *(please note that the quality of teaching hospitals vastly differ between Uganda and the United States)*. The remaining elective and core rotations are undertaken at Pineville Community Hospital in Kentucky. At the moment, the medical school is actively searching to establish other clinical sites in the US and England.

Note: Kigezi International also offers a five-year M.D. program for non-traditional applicants who have not completed the pre-medical requirements, and for applicants without a prior degree.

The Campus

While in Cambridge, students have the privilege of attending seminars and concerts held within the University of Cambridge colleges. Living at Westminster College affords the students a taste of the traditional Cambridge experience. The academic calender of the medical program follows the Cambridge trimester system. It is important to note that at no time are students in Kigezi's medical program officially members of Cambridge University. However, students do enjoy the benefits of Cambridge's student life. Most cultural and social events sponsored by the thirty-three colleges of Cambridge are open to Kigezi's medical students.

Students live in rooms of one of two sizes. The smaller rooms are priced at £35 per week, while the larger rooms cost £45 per week. The carpeted rooms are furnished with a bed, desk, chair, and a chest of drawers. The larger rooms are furnished with a few other items. However, students share kitchens and bathroom facilities. Shops and restaurants in the city center are within walking distance from the living quarters.

Financial Aid

All tuition and housing fees for each term must be paid no later than one month before the start of the term.

U.S. citizens and green-card holders admitted to Kigezi International School of Medicine are not eligible for U.S. Federal Loan programs including the Stafford Loan. At this point, the school does not offer any comprehensive financial aid package. However, the Hansing Merit Scholarships (grants up to £5000 [approx. $7000]) are awarded to a few deserving students. Recipients of the Hansing Scholarship are chosen by members of the Directors of Admissions, and must maintain an exceptional academic record to be considered for renewal of the award each year.

For students who performs satisfactorily on USMLE I, Kigezi International offers a low interest loan to cover up to 50% of the cost of the clinical part of the curriculum.

Israel

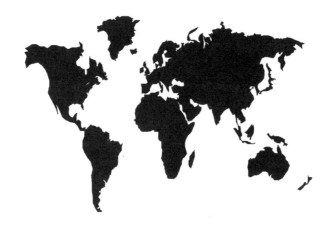

Touro College
Touro-Technion M.A./M.D. Program

Office of Admissions
Center for Biomedical Education
Touro College
135 Carman Road • Bldg #10
Dix Hills • N.Y. 11746
Phone: (516) 673-3200 ext. 222 • Fax: (516) 673-3432

The School Profile

Tuoro College is accredited by the Commission on Higher Education of the Middle States Association of Colleges and Schools. The M.D. degree program of the Faculty of Medicine of the Technion-Israel Institute of Technology is fully accredited by Israel's National Council for Higher Education and is listed in the Directory of Medical Schools of the WHO.

The Center for Biomedical Education of Touro College is located on the campus of the Long Island Developmental Center in Dix Hills. Within the developmental center, Touro College occupies buildings 10 and 14. Classrooms, laboratories, the college library, dining rooms, and administrative offices are all located in these two buildings.

The Technion Faculty of Medicine is located in the B. Rappaport Family-Medical Sciences Building at Bat Galim, Haifa, Israel. The building is comprised of basic science research laboratories, the preclinical teaching departments, the central Medical School Library, and lecture halls. The Technion Faculty of Medicine serves as the primary center for the study and practice of medicine in the northern Israel region.

Location

Haifa is Israel's third largest city. Situated in a wide natural bay between the beautiful Mediterranean Sea and the Carmel mountain, the city's terraced landscape offers a rich variety of breathtaking panoramas, giving the observer the sensation of being on a heavenly peninsula. To the northeast, across the sparkling waters of the harbor, sits the medieval walled fortress city of Acre. Directly north, beckon the heights of Rosh Hanikra, the majestic white cliff. Further east towers the snow-capped peak of Mount Hermon. Haifa is traditional, contemporary, sophisticated and relaxed. Theaters, museums, movie theaters, elegant hotels, air-conditioned shopping malls and sandy beaches are abundant in Haifa.

Admission Requirements

The minimum admission requirements for applicants from North America (the United States and Canada) are the following:

- A bachelor's degree from an accredited university or college prior to matriculation into the University.
- Completion of premedical curriculum that includes the following courses:
    1. General biology with laboratory – one year (two semesters)
    2. Inorganic chemistry with laboratory – one year (two semesters)
    3. Organic chemistry with laboratory – one year (two semesters)
    4. Physics with laboratory – one year (two semesters)
    5. Mathematics (Calculus, computer science, or statistics) – strongly recommended
    6. English – one year (two semesters)
- Medical College Admission Test (MCAT) score

Selection Factors

According to the college brochure, "...applicants are evaluated first by the Admissions Committee of the Biomedical Sciences Department of Touro College as possible candidates for admissions...". Those applicants deemed to be qualified are invited for interviews with the members of the admissions committee. If accepted by the Touro admissions committee, applicants are re-invited for a second interview with the members of the admissions committee from the Technion. The candidates are notified of the Technion's decision within one week following the interview.

The Curriculum

The MA/MD track is designed for those individuals who wish to pursue a career as a physician. It combines the Master of Arts in Interdisciplinary Studies in Biological and Physical Sciences. A minimum of five years of study is required to complete the Touro/Technion joint program in medicine.

During the first year, all students complete the MA track at Touro. The credits earned at Touro are then accepted for advanced standing at the Technion, where an additional four years of study are required for the MD degree. A submission of thesis is also required for successful graduation from the program.

Clinical education takes place in the formally accredited affiliated hospitals Rambam, Haifa Medical Center, and Carmel (all located in Haifa) and in affiliated institutions in Nahariya, Afula, and Safed, Israel.

Tuition & Fees

■ *Tuition for the MA/MD Track at Touro College*

Year One
Fall Semester $7,500
Spring Semester $7,500
Summer Semester $2,000

■ *Tuition at the Technion Faculty of Medicine, Israel*

Year Two $17,100
Year Three $17,100
Year Four $17,100
Year Five   no tuition

■ *Fees:*

Application Fee $75
Administration Fee $100 per semester
Graduation Fee $150
Microscope Rental $200 at Touro/$400 at the Technion
Books   Approximately $500-$1000 per year

Financial Aid

U.S. citizens may apply for Federal Government student loans such as the Stafford Loan to finance their medical education.

India

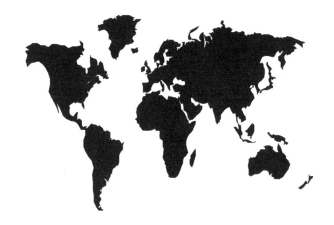

Jawaharlal Nehru Medical College
Belgaum

Belgaum • Karnataka • India
Phone: 011-91-831-451350 • Fax: 011-91-831-420782

Dr. D. P. Shetru
3210 Bloomfield Lane • Auburn Hills • MI 48326
Phone: (810) 852-6897

The School Profile

The Jawarhal Nehru Medical College was established in 1963 under the direction of K.L.E. Society and the State Government of Karnataka. The Medical College was recognized by both Karnataka University and the Medical Council of India in 1976.

The college is located on a 100 acre campus in Belgaum, Karnataka. The campus is comprised of a main building, library, dormitories for males and females and sports facilities. In addition, a spacious auditorium, a bank, a post office and a communication center are also located on-campus. In recent years, the Medical College has made rapid progress in its academic and research activities. The College offers both graduate and post-graduate programs in various medical disciplines.

The studentbody at the Jawaharlal Nehru Medical College hails primarily from India. However, students from the United States, Canada, the United Kingdom, the Middle East and Africa also attend the medical college.

Location

Belgaum is located in the northern part of the Indian state of Karnaraka. The city enjoys a temperate to hot climate throughout the year. During the summer the temperature ranges between 26°C and 34°C. The winters are pleasant and sunny.

Belgaum is on the Poona-Bangalore National Highway, connected by trains and airplanes to the rest of India.   The city is cosmopolitan in nature since it is comprised of the mixed cultures of Karnataka and Maharashtra (neighboring Indian state).

Admission Requirements

The minimum admission requirements for applicants from North America (the United States and Canada) are the following:

- A bachelor's degree from an accredited university or college or High School diploma.

- Completion of college or high school curriculum that includes the following courses:
    1. General biology with laboratory
    2. Inorganic chemistry with laboratory
    3. Organic chemistry with laboratory
    4. Physics with laboratory

- Medical College Admission Test (MCAT) score not required.

- The applicant must be at least 17 years of age.

Selection Factors

Information Not Available.

The Curriculum

The medical curriculum of Jawaharlal Nehru Medical College is four and a half years long . The curriculum is comprised of traditional medical education followed by a year of compulsory rotating internships.

Jawaharlal Nehru Medical College grants the medical degree of MBBS following the successful completion of the following curriculum:

MBBS Phase I courses (Pre-Clinical) – 1½ years long
1. Anatomy
2. Physiology
3. Biochemistry
4. Community Medicine

MBBS Phase II courses (Para Clinical) – 1½ years long
1. Pharmacology
2. Pathology
3. Microbiology
4. Forensic Medicine

MBBS Pase III (Clinical) – 1½ years long

Teaching Facilities

Didactic teaching related to basic sciences is conducted in the main building located within the 100 acre college campus. Students complete their pre-clinical courses within the confines of this building. In addition to classrooms, the main building also houses various laboratories for student use.

The K.L.E. Society's Hospital & Medical Research Center and the Government District Hospital serve as teaching hospitals. The clinical trainings are conducted in both of these hospitals under the guidance of the hospital staff.

Financial Aid

U.S. citizens enrolled full-time at Jawaharlal Nehru Medical College are **not** eligible for Federal Student Loan Programs. Information related to other forms of financial aid packages was not available.

Australia

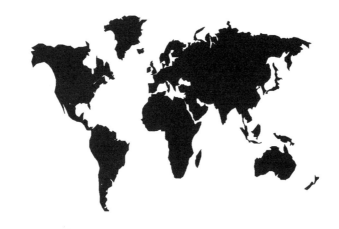

Flinders University
Faculty of Health Sciences

International Office • GPO Box 2100
Adelaide SA 5001 • Australia
Phone: 1-800-686-3562 • 011-61-618-201-2727
Fax: 011-61-618-201-3177
Internet: http://som.flinders.edu.au/

The School Profile

The Flinders University of South Australia was founded in 1966. It was named after the explorer, Mathew Flinders, who in 1802, was the first European to sail along the coast of St. Vincent Gulf. Flinders is a modern university with an international reputation for excellence in teaching and research. The University supports a teaching staff of over 700 professors. Flinders is funded by the Government and is a member of the Association of Commonwealth Universities.

The University's Faculty of Health Sciences include the medical school. The Medical School was established in 1975 and since then it has trained many physicians. In addition to training new physicians, the medical school also offers training in the areas of nutrition and dietetics, public and environmental health, speech pathology, cognitive science and biotechnology.

Flinders University's student body is comprised of more than 10,000 students. Approximately 10% of the students on-campus are foreign.

Location

Adelaide is the capital of the state of South Australia. It is a cosmopolitan city of approximately one million people and is the chief commercial, cultural and administrative center of the State.

Founded in 1836 by Col. William Light, Adelaide is the only capital to have been established by free settlers. Surrounded by miles of white sandy beaches, Adelaide is ideally located as a center for the marine sciences. The city's coastline offers swimming, diving, sailing, fishing and other water sports. The city is also home to Australia's many cultural activities. It is renown for its thriving arts scene and an international biennial arts festival. The city also features one of Australia's most significant public art galleries, the Art Gallery of South Australia.

Adelaide enjoys a wide range of restaurants, bistros and side-walk cafes throughout the city. Places of worship of most faiths are available in the city. Adelaide also boasts an efficient public transport system of regular bus, train and tram services. Flinders University is accessible by public

Admission Requirements

The minimum admission requirements for applicants from North America (the United States and Canada) are as follows:

- A bachelor's degree from an accredited university or college or High School diploma.

- There are no specific university courses which must be have been completed before an application is filed with the University.

- Medical College Admission Test (MCAT) score is required. The MCAT score cannot be more than two years old.

Selection Factors

The three elements that contribute to selection for admission are as follows:

- Performance in undergraduate courses
- The MCAT score
- Personal Admissions Interview

Undergraduate Degree – Applicants must have performed at a high academic level in an undergraduate degree granting program. A weighted GPA is calculated based on an applicant's undergraduate performance. It is expected that successful applicants will have a B or better average. Greater weight is given to an applicant's performance in later years.

MCAT – Applicants are required to achieve a minimum standard in each section of the MCAT. The overall score from the MCAT is used to identify applicants for a personal interview and final ranking.

Personal Interview – Applicants are compared on the basis of undergraduate GPA and MCAT scores. The best applicants are invited for an in-person interview, to assess personal qualities and proficiency in spoken English.

Final Ranking – The final ranking of applicants is based on a combination of a weighted GPA, MCAT score and the interview.

The Curriculum

The new four-year medical program at Flinders is founded on problem-based learning. Students learn medicine in a framework similar to that in which doctors practice, to help prepare them for a process of learning and professional development that will continue throughout their lives as medical practitioners.

Formal lectures are kept to a minimum. Instead, students take an active role in assembling, evaluating and applying the knowledge necessary to define and solve each problem. The problem-based framework allows the integration of the basic medical sciences and social perspectives with clinical medicine throughout the curriculum.

In Years one and two, the problems which provide the focus for student learning are grouped into blocks dealing with principles of human biology. Within each block, clinical skills tutorials teach the interpersonal and procedural skills important in establishing an effective relationship between doctor and patient.

In Years three and four, students work with physicians to complete the clinical part of the curriculum at university affiliated hospitals. Through a series of rotations in key areas of medicine, students acquire a broad experience in healthcare.

The Campus

Flinders University is situated approximately 6 miles from the center of Adelaide in the southern foothills of the Mt. Lofty Ranges. Since the University was established in 1966, it has expanded rapidly to include the teaching facilities of a major public hospital, the adjacent Flinders Medical Center, and the former Sturt Campus of the South Amustralian College of Advanced Education.

The large campus is one of Australia's most beautiful campuses. The campus is characterized by modern academic buildings situated amongst natural bushland, a pine forest, gardens, a tree-fringed lake and sweeping lawns.

Financial Aid

Flinders University does not offer scholarships for students studying medicine. Australian Government scholarships may be available to students from some countries. U.S. citizens may apply for Federal loans such as the Stafford Loan to finance their medical education.

Note from the Publisher: Beginning in 1997, Flinders University along with Sydney and Queensland Universities, will offer foreign residents (including U.S. citizens) a chance to enroll in their four-year medical program.

Flinders, Sydney and Queensland Universities will together offer 60 places for enrollment to international students.

More Foreign Medical Schools
Selected Regions

PAKISTAN

The Aga Khan University Medical College

The Admissions Office
P.O. Box 3500
Stadium Road
Karachi 74800
Pakistan

Telephone# (92) 21-493-0051
Fax# (92) 21-493-4294

Internet: http://www.cybercom.net/~jafary/ (Unofficial Web Site)

Admissions Requirements:
High School Diploma and Achievement Test score of 600 or above in biology, chemistry and physics or mathematics.

SAT (minimum score of 1100) or MCAT (minimum score of 24)

Sindh Medical College

Contact Arif Khalil Mirza (Class of 2000) for more information on Sindh Medical College.

Unofficial Web Site: http://kolachi.com/smc
E-mail address: akm@paknet3.ptc.pk

PHILIPPINES

University of the East
Ramon Magsaysay Memorial Medical Center

UERM University Registrar
UERMMMC College of Medicine
Aurora Blvd.
Quezon City
Philippines

Dr. Felicidad Soto – Chairperson of Admissions Committee
cerebrum@mnl.sequel.net (you can contact Dr. Soto at this e-mail address).

Telephone#
(Country code of Philippines) + (Quezon City code) + 713-3315
Fax#
(Country code of Philippines) + (Quezon City code) + 715-1070

Internet: http://www.sequel.net/~fpi/tips.html
    *Tips from current U.S. citizens attending UERMMMC are posted
    at the site.*

Admissions Requirements:
NMAT Score
Contact the University Registrar for NMAT information. You can also contact
the nearest Philippine Consulate in major U.S. cities for NMAT information.
The NMAT is offered in Los Angeles and New York twice a year.

IRELAND

Royal College of Surgeon
Dublin, Ireland

The Atlantic Bridge Program
*The only English-speaking European medical school that accepts U.S.
citizens.*

Telephone# 1-800-876-3876

Fax# 714-723-6318

What's On The Net?

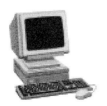

The explosion of web sites on the Internet has been a boon for everyone who is seeking admission to medical school. A wealth of information ranging from the application process to residency matches is now available on the net. It is important that every decision you make regarding your future profession be an informed decision.

The key to finding the information you want on the Internet is persistence. The most effective way to find information on the net is to use the proper "search" words when using search engines like Yahoo, Alta Vista or Excite. Another effective search technique is to find web sites with links to similar sites on the World Wide Web or the Internet. Increasingly, medical information web designers are doing a commendable job of linking content-similar web sites to their own sites.

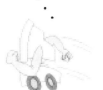

On the next few pages, you will find home page addresses and brief descriptions of web sites that are pre-med student friendly. At these sites, you will find important facts and information that will help you learn more about medical schools and the "mysterious" admission process.

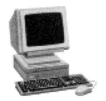

Key Search Words for the Internet

Use the following words to find foreign medical school related web sites on the net:

foreign medical schools

foreign medical graduates

international medical schools

ECFMG

USMLE

Caribbean medical schools

European medical schools

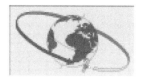

...Connecting to the Internet

Searching for Medical Web Sites...

Medical School Web Sites

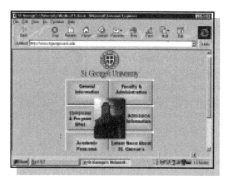

St. Georges's University
School of Medicine

http://www.stgeorgesuniv.edu

The official web site of St. George's University. You will find all the information you need regarding the School of Medicine.

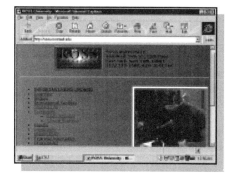

Ross University
School of Medicine

http://www.rossmed.edu

The official web site of Ross University School of Medicine. Everything you need to know about the admissions process is right here.

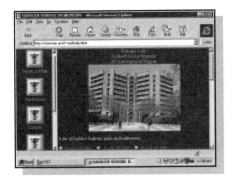

Sackler
School of Medicine

http://www.tau.ac.il/~ori/body.html

The official web site of Sackler School of Medicine. This site is full of information, with links to student e-mail addresses and more.

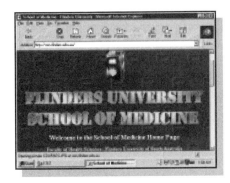

Flinders University
School of Medicine

http://som.flinders.edu.au/

The official web site of Flinders University School of Medicine. This web site provides valuable information, including a discussion of the application process, at this Australian medical school.

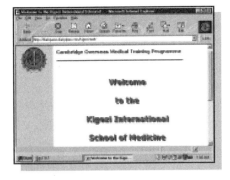

Kigezi International
School of Medicine

*http://dialspace.dial.pipex.com/
kigezi.med/*

The official web site of Cambridge Overseas Medical Training Program. Learn more about Kigezi's medical curriculum at this site.

Other Helpful Web Sites on the Internet

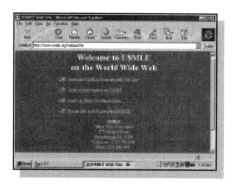

United States Medical Licensing Examination (USMLE)

http://www.usmle.org

The ultimate USMLE home page. Learn more about the USMLE test at this information saturated web site.

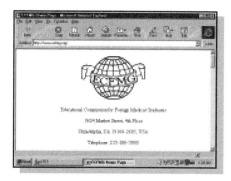

ECFMG

http://www.ecfmg.org

Learn more about the certification process all foreign medical graduates (U.S. or non-U.S. citizens) must go through in order to obtain a medical license in the United States.

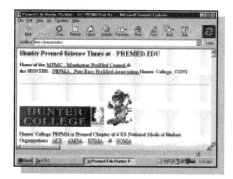

Hunter College Pre-Med Home Page

http://premed.edu/

A great web site for all premeds. You will find lots of information and many links to other similar web sites. A must see site for anyone interested in attending medical school.

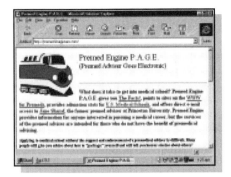

Premed Engine P.A.G.E.
Premed Adviser Goes Electronic

http://premed.imagiware.com/

This web site is maintained by Jane Sharaf, the former premed adviser at Princeton University. A wealth of information on what it takes to get into medical schools can be found at this site.

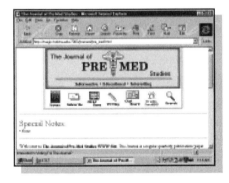

The Journal of Pre-Med Studies

http://magic.hofstra.edu:7003/ premed/pre_med.html

The official web site of The Journal of Pre-Med Studies. A well-organized site that explores numerous aspects of pre-medical education. Another must see site!

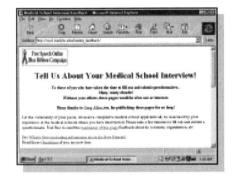

Medical School Interview
Feedback Home Page

http://ww2.med.jhu.edu/ meded_feedback/

This web site publishes feedbacks from students who have been interviewed by medical schools. It's worth your time to check out what's on this site.

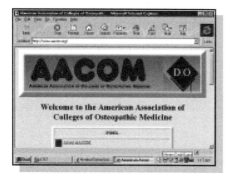

American Association of Colleges of Osteopathic Medicine

http://www.aacom.org

If you are interested in attending osteopathic medical school (D.O. degree), this is the web site for you.

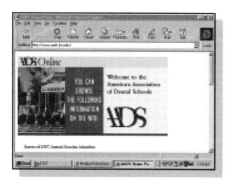

American Association of Dental Schools

http://www.aads.jhu.edu/

The official web site of AADS. If your dream is to become a dentist, don't miss this site. Learn about the dental school application process.

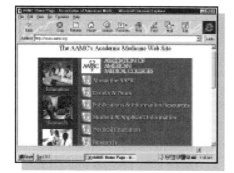

Association of American Medical Colleges

http://www.aamc.org

The official web site of American medical colleges. AMCAS application may be downloaded from this site. The mecca of all medical school sites.

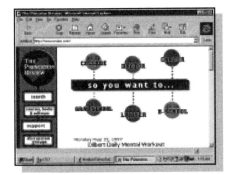

The Princeton Review

http://www.review.com

The official web site of one of the leading test-prep companies in the U.S. You will find a wide range of information and facts related to the college admissions process and standardized tests at this site.

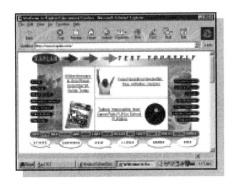

KAPLAN

http://www.kaplan.com

Another great web site dedicated to the college admissions process and standardized tests. The official web site of Kaplan, a leading test-prep company, is well worth a visit.

International Medical Schools

The Complete List

List Of
International Medical Schools

Australia

• John Curtin School of Medical Science at the Australian National University
• Monash University Medical Informatics
• University of Adelaide
• University of Sydney
• University of Queensland

Belgium

• Vrije Universiteit Brussel, Faculteit Geneeskunde en Farmacie

Brazil

• Hospital da Faculdade de Medicina de Botucatu - UNESP - Brazil

Canada

• McGill University - Medical Computing Resource
• M.I.R. University of Calgary
• University of British Columbia

China

• Shanghai Medical University

Czech Republic

• Charles University

Denmark

• University of Copenhagen Information

Finland

• University of Oulo, faculty of Medicine
• University of Turku, Faculty of Medicine

Germany

• RWTH Aachen
• Freie Universität Berlin
• Universität Bonn
• Universität Düsseldorf: Medizinische Fakultät
• Universität Erlangen
• Universität Frankfurt
• Universität Göttingen, Fachbereich Medizin
• Universität Hamburg
• Universität Heidelberg
• Universität Jena
• Universität Köln
• Universität Leipzig
• Universität Lübeck
• Universität München
• Universität Münster
• Universität Rostock
• Universität Ulm

Hungary

- Albert Szent-Györgyi Medical University, Szeged
- Semmelweis University of Medical Sciences
- University Medical School of Medicine, Debrecen

Israel

- Ben Gurion University of the Negev Faculty of Health Sciences
- The Hebrew University - Hadassah Medical School
- Sackler School of Medicine, Tel Aviv University

Japan

- Mie University School of Medicine
- Miyazaki Medical College
- Nagoya University Medical School
- Osaka Medical School
- Sapporo Medical School
- School of Medicine, Kyoto University
- School of Medicine, Mie University
- School of Medicine, Nagoya University
- School of Medicine, Nippon University
- Nippon Medical School
- Osaka Medical College
- School of Medicine, Tokushima University
- Shiga University of Medical Science

The Netherlands

- Erasmus University, Rotterdam
- University of Limburg, Maastricht

Norway

- University of Oslo, Norway, Faculty of Medicine
- University of Bergen, Norway, Faculty of Medicine

• University of Tromsø, Norway, Faculty of Medicine
• University of Trondheim, Norway, Faculty of Medicine

Poland

• Gdansk Medical Academy
• Lodz Medical Academy
• Poznan Medical Academy

Singapore

• National University of Singapore (NUS), Faculty of Medicine

South Africa

• Faculty of Medicine, University of CapeTown

Sweden

• Karolinska Institute
• Uppsala University: Departments
• Medicinsk Fakultet, Umeå
• Medicinska fakulteten, GU(Göteborg)
• Lund University

Taiwan

• China Medical College

The United Kingdom

• London Royal Free Hospital School of Medicine
• Royal Postgraduate Medical School
• United Medical and Dental School of Guys and St Thomas's Hospitals

Wales

• Institute for Health Informatics, University of Wales, Aberystwyth

Facts, Facts, and More Facts

More Info You *Need* To Know

Facts, Facts, and More Facts ...Info You Can Use

U.S. allopathic and osteopathic medical school statistics

Information you are dying to know!

LIST OF OSTEOPATHIC MEDICAL SCHOOLS

D.O. Degree Granting Schools

1996 Entering Class Data

Arizona College of Osteopathic Medicine of Midwestern University
(AZCOM)
19555 N. 59th Avenue
Glendale, ARIZONA 85308
(708) 515-6472

Chicago College of Osteopathic Medicine of Midwestern
University (CCOM)
555 31st Street
Downers Grove, Illinois 60515-1235
(708) 515-6472
Average MCAT: 8.4
Average GPA: 3.4
In State: 51% Class Size: 150

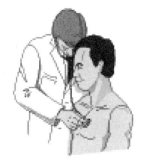

Kirksville College of Osteopathic Medicine (KCOM)
800 West Jefferson Street
Kirksville, Missouri 63501
(816) 626-2121
Average MCAT: 8.6
Average GPA: 3.3
In State: 14% Class Size: 145

Lake Erie College of Osteopathic Medicine (LECOM)
1858 W. Grandview Boulevard
Erie, Pennsylvania 16509
(814) 866-6565
Average MCAT: 7.2
Average GPA: 3.1
In State: 48% Class Size: 100

Michigan State University College of Osteopathic Medicine (MSU-COM)
East Lansing, Michigan 48824
(517) 355-9611
Average MCAT: 8.0
Average GPA: 3.4
In State: 84% Class Size: 125

New York College of Osteopathic Medicine of New York Institute of
Technology (NYCOM)
Wheatley Road, Box 170
Old Westbury, New York 11568
(516) 626-6900
Average MCAT: 7.3
Average GPA: 3.2
In State: 79% Class Size: 180

Nova Southeastern University Health Professions Division College of
Osteopathic Medicine (NSUCOM)
3200 S. University Drive
Fort Lauderdale, Florida 33328
(954) 723-1000
Average MCAT: 8.0
Average GPA: 3.4
In State: 56% Class Size: 150

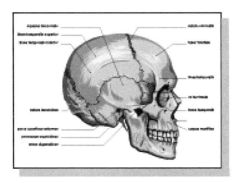

Ohio University College of Osteopathic Medicine
(OUCOM)
Grosvenor and Irvine Halls
Athens, Ohio 45701
(614) 593-2500
Average MCAT: 8.2
Average GPA: 3.4
In State: 66% Class Size: 100

Oklahoma State University College of Osteopathic Medicine (OSU/COM)
1111 West 17th Street
Tulsa, Oklahoma 74107
(918) 582-1972
Average MCAT: 8.2
Average GPA: 3.4
In State: 81% Class Size: 88

Philadelphia College of Osteopathic Medicine (PCOM)
4170 City Avenue
Philadelphia, Pennsylvania 19131
(215) 871-1000
Average MCAT: 7.9
Average GPA: 3.3
In State: 70% Class Size: 250

The University of Health Sciences-College of Osteopathic Medicine
(UHS-COM)
2105 Independence Boulevard
Kansas City, Missouri 64124
(816) 283-2000
Average MCAT: 7.7
Average GPA: 3.3
In State: 20% Class Size: 180

University of Medicine and Dentistry of New Jersey School of
Osteopathic Medicine (UMDNJ-SOM)
One Medical Center Drive, Suite 312
Stratford, New Jersey 08084
(609) 566-6990
Average MCAT: 8.0
Average GPA: 3.5
In State: 91% Class Size: 75

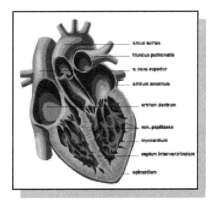

University of New England College of Osteopathic
Medicine (UNECOM)
11 Hills Beach Road
Biddeford, Maine 04005
(207) 283-0171
Average MCAT: 7.5
Average GPA: 3.2
In State: 17% Class Size: 80

University of North Texas Health Science Center at Fort Worth - Texas
College of Osteopathic Medicine (UNTHSC)
3500 Camp Bowie Boulevard
Fort Worth, Texas 76107
(817) 735-2000
Average MCAT: 8.4
Average GPA: 3.4
In State: 94% Class Size: 100

University of Osteopathic Medicine and Health Sciences
3200 Grand Avenue
Des Moines, Iowa 50312
(515) 271-1400
Average MCAT: 8.1
Average GPA: 3.3
In State: 17% Class Size: 205

West Virginia School of Osteopathic Medicine (WVSOM)
400 North Lee Street
Lewisburg, West Virginia 24901
(304) 645-6270
Average MCAT: NA
Average GPA: 3.5
In State: 70% Class Size: 65

Western University of the Health Sciences, College of Osteopathic
Medicine of the Pacific (COMP)
College Plaza
Pomona, California 91766-1889
(909) 623-6116
Average MCAT: 8.2
Average GPA: 3.2
In State: 72% Class Size: 176

Source: Osteopathic Medical College Information,
1996 Entering Class.

Average MCAT and GPAs at U.S. Medical Schools

University of Alabama at Birmingham
Average MCAT: 9.7
Average GPA: 3.6

University of South Alabama
Average MCAT: 9.3
Average GPA: 3.6

University of Arizona
Average MCAT: 9.4
Average GPA: 3.5

University of Arkansas
Average MCAT: 7.6
Average GPA: 3.5

Loma Linda University
Average MCAT: 8.9
Average GPA: 3.6

Stanford University
Average MCAT: 10.8
Average GPA: 3.6

University of California - Davis
Average MCAT: 11.0
Average GPA: 3.5

University of California - Irvine
Average MCAT: 10.2
Average GPA: 3.

University of California - Los Angeles
Average MCAT: 10.5
Average GPA: 3.6

University of California - San Diego
Average MCAT: 11.0
Average GPA: 3.6

University of California - San Francisco
Average MCAT: 11.0
Average GPA: 3.7

University of Southern California
Average MCAT: 10.0
Average GPA: 3.5

University of Colorado
Average MCAT: 9.9
Average GPA: 3.7

University of Connecticut
Average MCAT: 9.7
Average GPA: 3.5

Yale University
Average MCAT: 11.0
Average GPA: 3.6

George Washington University
Average MCAT: 9.4
Average GPA: 3.5

Georgetown University
Average MCAT: 10.0
Average GPA: 3.5

Howard University
Average MCAT: 7.0
Average GPA: 3.0

University of Florida
Average MCAT: 9.3
Average GPA: 3.7

University of Miami
Average MCAT: 9.4
Average GPA: 3.6

University of South Florida
Average MCAT: 9.7
Average GPA: 3.7

Emory University
Average MCAT: 9.8
Average GPA: 3.6.

Medical College of Georgia
Average MCAT: 9.4
Average GPA: 3.5

Mercer University
Average MCAT: 8.6
Average GPA: 3.3

Morehouse School of Medicine
Average MCAT: 7.0
Average GPA: 3.0

University of Hawaii
Average MCAT: 9.5
Average GPA: 3.4

Chicago Medical School, Finch University for
Health Sciences
Average MCAT: 9.0
Average GPA: 3.2

Loyola University of Chicago Stritch
Average MCAT: 9.5
Average GPA: 3.5

Northwestern University
Average MCAT: 9.7
Average GPA: 3.5

Rush University
Average MCAT: 9.1
Average GPA: 3.4

Southern Illinois University at Springfield
Average MCAT: 8.8
Average GPA: 3.5

University of Chicago Pritzker School of
Medicine
Average MCAT: 10.2
Average GPA: 3.5

University of Illinois at Chicago
Average MCAT: 9.3
Average GPA: 3.4

Indiana University at Indianapolis
Average MCAT: 9.4
Average GPA: 3.6

University of Iowa
Average MCAT: 9.4
Average GPA: 3.6

University of Kansas
Average MCAT: 9.1
Average GPA: 3.5

University of Kentucky
Average MCAT: 9.0
Average GPA: 3.44

University of Louisville
Average MCAT: 8.9
Average GPA: 3.4

Louisiana State University - New Orleans
Average MCAT: 8.6
Average GPA: 3.4

Louisiana State University - Shreveport
Average MCAT: 8.8
Average GPA: 3.4

Tulane University
Average MCAT: 9.5
Average GPA: 3.5

Johns Hopkins University
Average MCAT: 11.0
Average GPA: 3.7

Uniformed Services University of the Health
Sciences
Average MCAT: 9.8
Average GPA: 3.4

University of Maryland at Baltimore
Average MCAT: 9.8
Average GPA: 3.6

Boston University
Average MCAT: 9.1
Average GPA: 3.3

Harvard University
Average MCAT: 11.0
Average GPA: 3.7

Tufts University
Average MCAT: 9.2
Average GPA: 3.5

University of Massachusetts at Worcester
Average MCAT: 10.0
Average GPA: 3.5

Michigan State University
Average MCAT: 9.3
Average GPA: 3.4

University of Michigan - Ann Arbor
Average MCAT: 10.7
Average GPA: 3.6

Wayne State University
Average MCAT: 8.9
Average GPA: 3.4

Mayo Medical School
Average MCAT: 10.7
Average GPA: 3.6

University of Minnesota - Duluth
Average MCAT: 8.9
Average GPA: 3.5

University of Minnesota - Minneapolis
Average MCAT: 9.7
Average GPA: 3.6

University of Mississippi
Average MCAT: 9.0
Average GPA: 3.6

St. Louis University
Average MCAT: 9.9
Average GPA: 3.6

University of Missouri - Columbia
Average MCAT: 9.3
Average GPA: 3.6

University of Missouri - Kansas City
Average MCAT: 8.0
Average GPA: 3.0

Washington University
Average MCAT: 11.4
Average GPA: 3.8

Creighton University
Average MCAT: 8.8
Average GPA: 3.6

University of Nebraska
Average MCAT: 9.2
Average GPA: 3.6

University of Nevada
Average MCAT: 9.2
Average GPA: 3.4

Dartmouth Medical School
Average MCAT: 9.6
Average GPA: 3.5

UMDNJ New Jersey Medical School
Average MCAT: 9.6
Average GPA: 3.3

UMDNJ Robert Wood Johnson Medical School
Average MCAT: 9.4
Average GPA: 3.5

University of New Mexico
Average MCAT: 8.9
Average GPA: 3.5

Albany Medical College
Average MCAT: 9.9
Average GPA: 3.4

Albert Einstein College of Medicine,
Yeshiva University
Average MCAT: 10.0
Average GPA: 3.5

Columbia University
Average MCAT: 10.7
Average GPA: 3.5

Cornell University
Average MCAT: 10.5
Average GPA: 3.5

Mount Sinai School of Medicine
Average MCAT: 9.1
Average GPA: 3.4

New York Medical College
Average MCAT: 10.0
Average GPA: 3.3

New York University
Average MCAT: 10.7
Average GPA: 3.6

SUNY - Brooklyn
Average MCAT: 9.3
Average GPA: 3.5

SUNY - Buffalo
Average MCAT: 9.6
Average GPA: 3.6

SUNY - Stony Brook
Average MCAT: 10.0
Average GPA: 3.5

SUNY - Syracuse
Average MCAT: 9.1
Average GPA: 3.5

University of Rochester
Average MCAT: 8.8
Average GPA: 3.5

Bowman Gray School of Medicine,
Wake Forest University
Average MCAT: 9.7
Average GPA: 3.4

Duke University
Average MCAT: 10.8
Average GPA: 3.6

East Carolina University
Average MCAT: 8.0
Average GPA: 3.4

University of North Carolina - Chapel Hill
Average MCAT: 9.0
Average GPA: 3.4

University of North Dakota
Average MCAT: 8.7
Average GPA: 3.6

Case Western Reserve University
Average MCAT: 9.5
Average GPA: 3.5

Medical College of Ohio
Average MCAT: 8.8
Average GPA: 3.4

Northeastern Ohio University
Average MCAT: 9.1
Average GPA: 3.6

Ohio State University
Average MCAT: 10.2
Average GPA: 3.6

University of Cincinnati
Average MCAT: 9.5
Average GPA: 3.5

Wright State University
Average MCAT: 8.0
Average GPA: 3.5

University of Oklahoma
Average MCAT: 9.2
Average GPA: 3.6

Oregon Health Sciences University
Average MCAT: 9.9
Average GPA: 3.6

Jefferson Medical College of
Thomas Jefferson University
Average MCAT: 9.5
Average GPA: 3.5

MCPHU Medical College of Pennsylvania and
Hahnemann University (MCP//HU)
Average MCAT: 10.0//9.2
Average GPA: 3.5//3.3

Pennsylvania State University
Average MCAT: 9.1
Average GPA: 3.5

Temple University
Average MCAT: 9.4
Average GPA: 3.3

University of Pennsylvania
Average MCAT: 10.7
Average GPA: 3.6

University of Pittsburgh
Average MCAT: 10.4
Average GPA: 3.5

Ponce School of Medicine
Average MCAT: 6.1
Average GPA: 3.3

Universidad del Caribe (in Bayamon, PR)
Average MCAT: 6.0
Average GPA: 3.1

University of Puerto Rico
Average MCAT: 7.0
Average GPA: 3.4

Brown University
Average MCAT: NA
Average GPA: 3.4

Medical University of South Carolina
Average MCAT: 9.0
Average GPA: 3.4

University of South Carolina
Average MCAT: 9.0
Average GPA: 3.4

University of South Dakota
Average MCAT: 8.5
Average GPA: 3.6

East Tennessee State University
Average MCAT: 8.7
Average GPA: 3.4

Meharry Medical College
Average MCAT: 7.5
Average GPA: 3.1

University of Tennessee at Memphis
Average MCAT: 9.0
Average GPA: 3.5

Vanderbilt University
Average MCAT: 11.0
Average GPA: 3.7

Baylor College of Medicine
Average MCAT: 10.3
Average GPA: 3.7

Texas A & M University
Average MCAT: 9.3
Average GPA: 3.5

Texas Tech University
Average MCAT: 9.3
Average GPA: 3.4

University of Texas,
Southwestern Medical School - Dallas
Average MCAT: 10.3
Average GPA: 3.6

University of Texas - Galveston
Average MCAT: 9.3
Average GPA: 3.5

University of Texas - Houston
Average MCAT: 8.7
Average GPA: 3.4

University of Texas - San Antonio
Average MCAT: 9.3
Average GPA: 3.6

University of Utah
Average MCAT: 10.5
Average GPA: 3.5

University of Vermont
Average MCAT: 8.9
Average GPA: 3.3

Eastern Virginia Medical School
Average MCAT: 9.0
Average GPA: 3.3

University of Virginia
Average MCAT: 10.2
Average GPA: 3.6

Virginia Commonwealth University
Medical College of Virginia
Average MCAT: 9.5
Average GPA: 3.3

University of Washington
Average MCAT: 10.0
Average GPA: 3.6

Marshall University
Average MCAT: 8.2
Average GPA: 3.5

West Virginia University
Average MCAT: 8.6
Average GPA: 3.6

Medical College of Wisconsin
Average MCAT: 9.0
Average GPA: 3.5

University of Wisconsin
Average MCAT: 9.5
Average GPA: 3.6

Sources: U.S. News & World Report, America's Best
Graduate Schools, 1995;
Association of American Medical Colleges, Medical School
Admission Requirements (MSAR), 1996-97

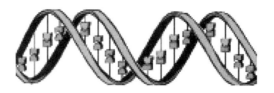

DNA – The Molecule of Life

Passing Rate of Foreign Medical School Graduates in USMLE I (U.S. & Foreign Citizens)

U.S. Citizens (Foreign Medical School Graduates)

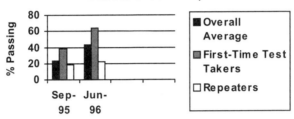

Foreign Citizens (Foreign Medical School Graduates)

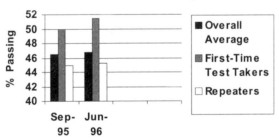

U.S. Medical Students

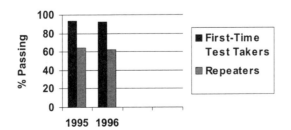

Appendix A

Application Checklist

■ Complete required premedical courses before or during the year you are applying to medical schools.

■ Meet with your university/college's premedical advisor.

■ Take the Medical College Admission Tests (MCAT) in April.

■ Obtain AMCAS application packet in late April/early May.

■ Obtain catalogs/brochures from foreign medical schools

■ Request professors to submit recommendation letters to your university/college's premedical advisor.

■ Request your premedical advisor to send the composite letter of recommendation to medical schools of your choice.

■ Contact graduates of and current students in U.S. and foreign medical schools for firsthand information on medical curriculums.

■ Attend informational seminars hosted by foreign medical schools at a city near you.

■ Track the progress of your applications once you have mailed them to various medical schools.

Appendix B

Medical School Inquiry Form

Medical School Inquiry Form		
School	Location	Date Catalog Requested

Appendix C

Application Tracking Form

Appendix D

Recommendation Letter Tracker

Letters of Recommendations

Recommender #1

Recommender's Name: _____

Recommender's Address: _____

_____

_____

Telephone Number: _____

Date Recommendation
Letter Mailed: _____

Recommender #2

Recommender's Name: _____

Recommender's Address: _____

_____

_____

Telephone Number: _____

Date Recommendation
Letter Mailed: _____

Recommender #3

Recommender's Name: _____

Recommender's Address: _____

_____

_____

Telephone Number: _____

Date Recommendation
Letter Mailed: _____

Recommender #4

Recommender's Name: _____

Recommender's Address: _____

_____

_____

Telephone Number: _____

Date Recommendation
Letter Mailed: _____

Appendix E

Interview Checklist

- Rule#1: BE YOURSELF!

- Be prepared.

- Review your application and the personal statement the night before your interview.

- Review the school's brochure.

- Prepare some questions about the medical curriculum for the interviewer.

- Sleep well the night before the interview.

- Arrive early to the interview site.

- Introduce yourself to the admission office staff and other intervieews.

- Take a deep breath and relax.

- Greet your interviewer(s) politely.

- Maintain eye contact with the interviewer.

- Concentrate and do not fidget with any items during the interview.

- Speak clearly and slowly.

- Respect your interviewer's professional status and avoid being arrogant.

- Maintain composure throughout the interview even when the interviewer is being antagonistic.

- Be truthful with your answers.

- Sincerely thank the interviewer for his or her time at the conclusion of the interview.

Appendix F

Typical Interview Questions

Personal Interest in Medicine Questions

- Why do you want to become a doctor?

- When did you decide that you wanted to pursue a career in medicine?

- What area of medicine are you interested in?

- Where do see yourself in ten years?

- Does the long working hours bother you?

- What do you like and dislike about medicine?

- The future of medicine is uncertain. Knowing that why do you want to enter the field of medicine?

- Do you think you are motivated enough to handle the rigors of medical school?

Holier than Thou Questions

- How would you feel treating an AIDS patient?

- What is your opinion regarding euthanasia?

- Would you work in a depressed area with indigent patients?

- What is your view of animal research?

- How do you think your role as a physician will affect society?

- Some people say doctors have the power to give or take life. How do you feel about "playing God"?

- What are the top three priorities of society?

Ex-patriot Questions

- Will you have any problems living in a country whose living standards are inferior to the American living standards?

- Do you have any particular dietary needs?

- Are you interested in learning about other cultures and people?

- Are you proficient in any foreign language?

- Do you have a fear of flying?

- Does warm, humid weather bother you?

- When you feel homesick, how will you deal with it?

- Can you afford to come here?

- What do you know about this country's history and political system?

- Have you ever lived anywhere outside the United States for an extensive period of time?

- Have you traveled to any foreign countries?

- What are some personal items that you plan to bring with you from the U.S. if you are accepted to this medical school?

- Do you mind living with roommates who may be from countries other than the United States?

MBA Questions

- Do you think health care is fast becoming unaffordable?

- Do you think doctors earn too much money?

- Do health insurance companies influence the way doctors practice medicine?

- How do you feel about socialized medicine?

- Describe what you believe to be the financial rewards of medicine.

- How will you finance your medical education?

Look into the Crystal Ball Questions

- What will be the biggest problem facing medicine in the future?

- Will managed care be the wave of the future?

- Do you think we will ever find a cure for AIDS or Cancer?

- How will you react the first time one of your patients dies?

Academic 101

- Why do you think you didn't do well on the MCAT?

- Explain your low organic chemistry grade?

- What was your favorite humanities course?

- Who was the author of your biochemistry book?

- Do you think you will succeed in medical school even though your overall GPA is low?

- Have you ever worked in a research laboratory?

- How have you improved your grades since you last applied to this school?

Tell Us About Yourself Questions

- What makes you angry?

- What is the biggest mistake you have ever made?

- What accomplishment are you most proud of?

- What are you hobbies?

- Tell me about your family.

- How do you deal with stress?

- Do you like being around sick people? Old people?

- How do you plan to deal with various professional prejudices that you may experience in the U.S. as a graduate of a foreign medical school?

- What five words best describe you?

- Are there any doctors in your family?

- Do you perceive yourself as a leader?

- What one event has affected you the most in the last five years?

- What did you do during the summers when you were in college?

- Is there someone you admire the most?

Mixed Bag Questions

- What is your favorite movie?

- Who is the Prime Minister of England?

- Do you know how to convert between miles and kilometers?

- Do you believe in drug legalization?

- Is there life after death?

- Who is your favorite basketball player?

- Do you believe racism still exists?

- What is the capital of Japan?

- What is your view regarding affirmative action?

- What is your opinion of current U.S. foreign policies?

- Do you have trouble working with different types of people?

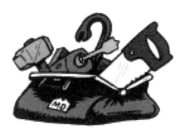

The Map Game

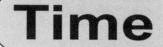

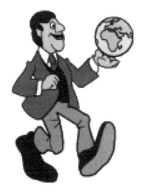

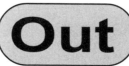

Time Out *for* FUN

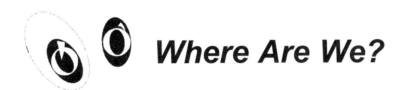 **Where Are We?**

Find the following European countries: Finland, France, Great Britain, Greece, Germany, Italy, Norway, Spain, Switzerland and the Netherlands

Your Answers:

A. _____

B. _____

C. _____

D. _____

E. _____

F. _____

G. _____

H. _____

I. _____

J. _____

North Sea

Atlantic Ocean

Mediterranean Sea

A B C D E F G H I J

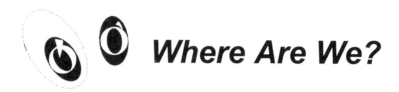

Where Are We?

Find the following Asian countries: Borneo, Burma, China, India, Iran, Mongolia and Saudi Arabia

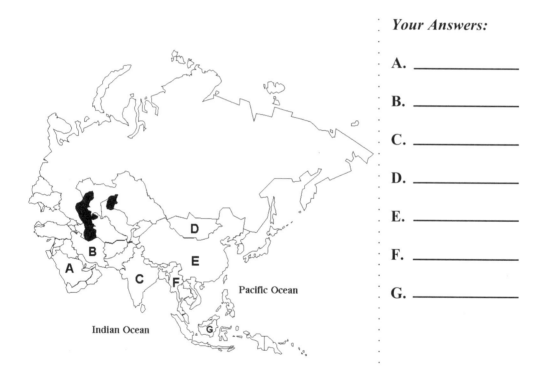

Your Answers:

A. _____

B. _____

C. _____

D. _____

E. _____

F. _____

G. _____

ANSWERS: **A.** *Saudi Arabia* **B.** *Iran* **C.** *India* **D.** *Mongolia* **E.** *China*
F. *Burma* **G.** *Borneo*

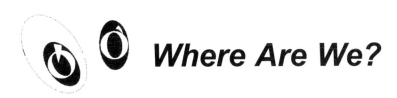

Where Are We?

Find the following American states: California, Florida,
Georgia, Illinois, Louisiana, Nebraska, New York, Ohio,
Texas and Washington

Your Answers:

A. _____

B. _____

C. _____

D. _____

E. _____

F. _____

G. _____

H. _____

I. _____

J. _____

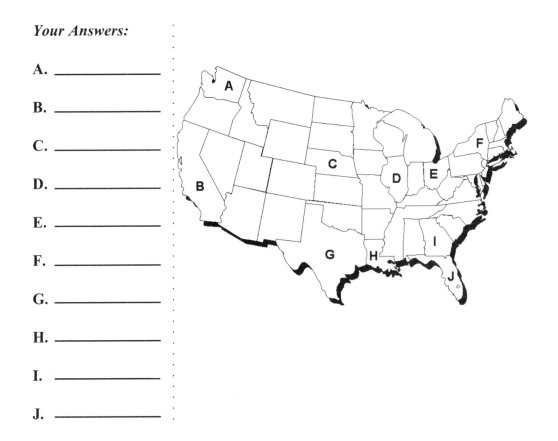

ANSWERS: **A.** *Washington* **B.** *California* **C.** *Nebraska* **D.** *Illinois* **E.** *Ohio*
F. *New York* **G.** *Texas* **H.** *Louisiana* I. *Georgia* J. *Florida*

Notes

Notes

Notes